CONTENTS

To Ali D, my rock
VF

To D, H and W
Thank you for sorting out all the symptoms I developed writing this book
KH

Symptom Sorter

FIFTH EDITION

Keith Hopcroft

and

Vincent Forte

General Practitioner
Central Surgery
Gorleston, Norfolk

Radcliffe Publishing
London • New York

Radcliffe Publishing Ltd
St Mark's House
Shepherdess Walk
London N1 7BQ
United Kingdom

www.radcliffehealth.com

© 2014 Keith Hopcroft and Vincent Forte

First Edition 1999
Second Edition 2003
Third Edition 2007
Fourth Edition 2010

Keith Hopcroft and Vincent Forte have asserted their right under the Copyright, Designs and Patents Act 1988 to be identified as the authors of this work.

Every effort has been made to ensure that the information in this book is accurate. This does not diminish the requirement to exercise clinical judgement, and neither the publisher nor the authors can accept any responsibility for its use in practice.

British Library Cataloguing in Publication Data

A catalogue record for this book is available from the British Library.

ISBN-13: 978 191022 718 3

The paper used for the text pages of this book is FSC certified. FSC (The Forest Stewardship Council) is an international network to promote responsible management of the world's forests.

Typeset by Darkriver Design, Auckland, New Zealand
Printed and bound by Hobbs the Printers, Totton, Hants, UK

ABBREVIATIONS

A&E	accident and emergency	DIC	disseminated intravascular coagulation
ABPI	ankle brachial pressure index		
ACE	angiotensin-converting enzyme	DKA	diabetic ketoacidosis
ACR	albumin creatinine ratio	DM	diabetes mellitus
ACTH	adrenocorticotrophic hormone	DU	duodenal ulcer
ADH	antidiuretic hormone	DUB	dysfunctional uterine bleeding
AF	atrial fibrillation	DVT	deep vein thrombosis
AFP	α fetoprotein	DXA	dual energy X-ray absorptiometry
ALT	alanine-amino transferase	EAM	external auditory meatus
ANUG	acute necrotising ulcerative gingivitis	EBV	Epstein–Barr virus
		ECG	electrocardiogram
ARC	AIDS-related complex	EEG	electroencephalogram
ASO	antistreptolysin	ELISA	enzyme-linked immunosorbent assay
AST	aspartate-amino transferase		
BCC	basal cell carcinoma	EMG	electromyography
BNP	B type natriuretic peptide	EMU	early morning urine (sample)
BP	blood pressure	ENT	ear, nose and throat
BPH	benign prostatic hypertrophy	EO	epididymo-orchitis
BTB	breakthrough bleeding	ERCP	endoscopic retrograde cholangiopancreaticogram
BV	bacterial vaginosis		
BXO	balanitis xerotica obliterans	ESR	erythrocyte sedimentation rate
CA-125	cancer antigen 125	ET	Eustachian tube
CCF	congestive cardiac failure	FBC	full blood count
CKD	chronic kidney disease	FSH	follicle-stimulating hormone
CNS	central nervous system	γGT	gamma glutamyl transpeptidase
COPD	chronic obstructive pulmonary disease	GAD	generalised anxiety disorder
		GF	glandular fever
CPK	creatine phosphokinase	GI	gastrointestinal
CREST	calcinosis/Raynaud's phenomenon/ oesophagealdysmotility/ sclerodactyly/telangiectasia	GI	granuloma inguinale
		GnRH	gonadotrophin-releasing hormone
		GORD	gastro-oesophageal reflux disease
CRF	chronic renal failure	GUM	genito-urinary medicine
CRP	C-reactive protein	Hb	haemoglobin
CSF	cerebrospinal fluid	HCG	human chorionic gonadotrophin
CT	carpal tunnel	5HIAA	5-hydroxy-indole-acetic acid
CT	computed tomography	HLA	human leucocyte antigen
CVA	cerebrovascular accident	HRT	hormone-replacement therapy
CXR	chest X-ray	HSV	herpes simplex virus
D&C	dilatation and curettage	HVS	high vaginal swab

IBD	inflammatory bowel disease	PEFR	peak expiratory flow rate
IBS	irritable bowel syndrome	PF	proctalgia fugax
IC	intermittent claudication	PID	pelvic inflammatory disease
IGTN	ingrowing toenail	PMR	polymyalgia rheumatica
IHD	ischaemic heart disease	PMT	pre-menstrual tension
INR	international normalised ratio	PR	per rectum
ITP	idiopathic thrombocytopenia purpura	PRIST	paper radioimmunosorbent disc test
IUCD	intrauterine contraceptive device	PSA	prostate-specific antigen
IVP	intravenous pyelogram	PTH	parathyroid hormone
IVU	intravenous urogram	PU	peptic ulcer
JCA	juvenile chronic arthritis	PUO	pyrexia of unknown origin
LFT	liver function tests	PV	per vagina
LGV	lymphogranuloma venereum	PVE	per vaginal examination
LH	luteinising hormone	PVD	peripheral vascular disease
LMP	last menstrual period	RA	rheumatoid arthritis
LN	lymph node	RAST	radioallergosorbent test
LRTI	lower respiratory tract infection	RAU	recurrent aphthous ulceration
LSD	lysergic acid diethylamide	RLS	restless legs syndrome
LUTS	lower urinary tract symptoms	RUQ	right upper quadrant
LVF	left ventricular failure	SA	septic arthritis
MAOI	monoamine oxidase inhibitor	SCC	squamous cell carcinoma
MC&S	microscopy, culture and sensitivity	SLE	systemic lupus erythematosus
MCV	mean cell volume	SOB	shortness of breath
MI	myocardial infarction	STD	sexually transmitted disease
MMR	measles, mumps, rubella	SVT	supraventricular tachycardia
MRI	magnetic resonance imaging	TAH	total abdominal hysterectomy
MS	multiple sclerosis	TATT	'tired all the time'
MSU	mid-stream urine (sample)	TB	tuberculosis
NAI	non-accidental injury	TCA	tricyclic antidepressant
NICE	National Institute for Health and Care Excellence	TFT	thyroid function tests
		TIA	transient ischaemic attack
NSAID	non-steroidal anti-inflammatory drug	TMJ	temporomandibular joint
		TN	trigeminal neuralgia
OA	osteoarthritis	TSH	thyroid-stimulating hormone
OE	otitis externa	TURP	transurethral resection of prostate
O/E	on examination	TV	trichomonal vaginosis
OG	onychogryphosis	U&E	urea and electrolytes
OGD	oesophago-gastro duodenoscopy	URTI	upper respiratory tract infection
OM	otitis media	UTI	urinary tract infection
OTC	over the counter	UV	ultraviolet
PAN	polyarteritis nodosa	VMA	vanillyl-mandelic acid
PCOS	polycystic ovary syndrome	V/Q	ventilation perfusion
PCR	protein creatinine ratio	VT	ventricular tachycardia
PCV	packed cell volume	WCC	white cell count
PE	pulmonary embolism	WRULD	work-related upper limb disorder

INTRODUCTION

Life would be much simpler for GPs if patients presented with diagnoses. Unfortunately, they do not: they present with symptoms, which are frequently vague, sometimes multiple and occasionally obscure. It is up to the GP to create some order from this chaos. However, the vast majority of clinical texts adopt a diagnosis, rather than symptom-based, approach and the few which do reflect the reality of patient presentations are inevitably orientated towards hospital medicine and so are irrelevant to GPs.

This book, originally serialised, in a different form, in *Doctor* magazine, aims to redress the balance. It analyses a multitude of symptoms commonly seen in primary care and, for each, presents differentials, distinguishing features, possible investigations and key points. The only omissions are presentations for which there are so few differentials that diagnosis is really quite simple (e.g. 'lump on elbow'); those which rarely present in isolation (e.g. nausea, anorexia); and those which are so rare that the reader would be sure to require specialist advice (our personal favourite being 'pilimiction').

Written by two full-time GP principals, its perspective is very much grass roots primary care – though informed by the latest evidence and guidance where possible or appropriate – and its appeal is therefore wide. GP registrars and young principals, relatively unfamiliar with the protean presentations possible in general practice, will be able to check their diagnostic hypotheses against the information in the book; the more experienced GP might use it as a refresher or as a pointer to a more exotic diagnosis in an unusual case; and the nurse practitioner, taking increasing responsibility as a first port of call in primary care for many patients, will find the contents unique and essential.

The popularity of the first edition and the need for second, third, fourth and fifth editions emphasises the fact that, while general practice may experience multiple reorganisations and restructurings, the bread and butter business of making sense of symptoms remains. This new edition adds a number of extra chapters and significant updates of existing chapters.

Each symptom is analysed in a uniform, accessible way, as follows.

The GP overview

This defines the symptom and its key characteristics, and gives some idea of the frequency of presentation.

Differential diagnosis

This lists the likely diagnoses, subdivided 'Common', 'Occasional' and 'Rare'. (It should be noted that these headings are relative to the symptom in question. For example, some of the 'common' causes of delayed puberty will be rarer than some of the 'occasional' causes of acute abdominal pain – for the simple reason that abdominal pain is much commoner than delayed puberty as a presenting symptom.) Restrictions of space and imagination mean that such a differential can never claim to be exhaustive, and a lack of accurate prevalence data renders the allocation of the diagnoses to these subdivisions somewhat arbitrary, based on our experience rather than hard evidence. These are minor limitations, however; this section will invariably provide clear guidance as to the likely cause of any symptom.

Ready reckoner

This provides a quick guide to the key distinguishing features of the five most likely diagnoses listed in the preceding section.

Possible investigations

This section outlines those investigations likely to assist the reader in making a diagnosis. The emphasis is upon tests performed in primary care or usually arranged by the GP. Where appropriate, more complex, hospital-initiated investigations are outlined – partly because GPs may wish to let their patients know the type of tests they might anticipate after referral and also because GP access to traditionally hospital-organised investigation is increasing. All investigations discussed are categorised according to the likelihood that they will be performed, the three categories being, 'Likely', 'Possible' and 'Small print'.

TOP TIPS

This provides a potpourri of management nuggets appropriate to each symptom, which the authors have accumulated over the years. Such hints from experience are difficult to analyse or quantify and so most are unashamedly anecdotal rather than evidence based – this should not detract from their usefulness or occasional elegance. Some might appear to stretch the scope of the book in that they cross the boundary between symptom assessment and symptom management – but the reader should bear in mind that the diagnostic process, particularly in primary care, involves hypothesis testing, and so these boundaries are, in reality, blurred.

Most symptoms presented in primary care are benign, minor and self-limiting. This can occasionally lull the unwary into a false sense of security: for each presentation there exist pointers which should set alarm bells ringing. 'Red flags' highlights aspects of symptoms which suggest significant pathology and which therefore should not be missed or neglected.

How to use this book

This *Symptom Sorter* is designed to act as a rapid reference. It has deliberately been written in a note and list format so that, unlike weightier tomes, it is quick and easy to use. For the sake of brevity, common and well-recognised abbreviations have been used whenever possible. Its consistent style will soon breed familiarity and allow the reader to know where and how to retrieve information painlessly. To help achieve this, the symptoms are arranged in sections, each section corresponding to a system or anatomical region. In these sections, the symptoms are arranged alphabetically and, for the most part, are labelled in patient, rather than doctor, vernacular (e.g. shortness of breath rather than dyspnoea) – the exceptions being where there is no acceptable or concise 'patientspeak' version. However, as many symptoms can have a variety of descriptions (e.g. shortness of breath, dyspnoea, breathlessness, wheeziness, difficulty breathing and so on) the index is deliberately expansive and cross-referenced, and will quickly guide the reader to the appropriate pages.

The categorisation of symptoms and their arrangement in sections is a complex task which can be approached in a number of ways – for example, rashes might be divided according to distribution, size of lesion, morphology, itch and so on. Throughout, we have chosen the approach which seems most logical to us and which, whenever possible, avoids unnecessary omission or repetition; again, the index should rapidly point the reader in the right direction. Assigning symptoms to certain sections may sometimes seem arbitrary, especially when they can have such disparate causes, but this approach provides the book with a clear, understandable structure.

As GPs, we are aware that patients often present polysymptomatically. Our book, neatly dividing complaints into individual symptoms, might therefore be criticised for not accurately reflecting real primary care life. In fact, such presentations can usually be distilled down to one or two predominant symptoms; more minor symptoms often act as pointers to the actual diagnosis, a fact our 'Ready reckoners' in each chapter exploits. In the truly polysymptomatic, the book may help to define a common thread among the symptoms, thereby revealing the real diagnosis – usually, in such cases, anxiety or depression.

The book should be kept to hand for use during surgery to confirm the likelihood of a certain diagnosis or raise the possibility of others. Being comprehensive, relevant and accessible, retrieval of information will be speedy and helpful during the consultation itself (you may wish to wait until the patient is undressing behind the curtain: there should be time).

The book may be used in other ways. GP trainers could use the analysis of a certain symptom provided in the text as the basis for a tutorial. Indeed, the book could itself form part of the GP registrar's curriculum. By 'sorting' two or three symptoms a week, using the text as a guide, the registrar could, over the course of his or her practice year, cover the vast majority of presentations seen in primary care. Trainers of undergraduates, too, will find that the contents provide useful material for teaching sessions.

Others might simply like to browse, refreshing or refining their diagnostic skills and mulling over the Red flags and Top tips.

Feedback received by the authors indicates that previous editions are now included in many undergraduate curricula as recommended reading, and the book is proving very popular among primary care nurses and nurse practitioners.

However the reader uses this book, we are convinced that it will prove an essential resource. Making sense of symptoms is the essence of general practice, and any tool designed by and for GPs which contributes to this art is likely to benefit doctors and patients alike.

Keith Hopcroft
Vincent Forte
August 2014

ABDOMEN

Abdominal swelling

Acute abdominal pain in adults

Acute abdominal pain in pregnancy

Chronic/recurrent abdominal pain in adults

Constipation

Diarrhoea

Epigastric pain

Recurrent childhood abdominal pain

Vomiting

Vomiting blood

ABDOMINAL SWELLING

The GP overview

This presentation covers both abdominal and pelvic masses, and general abdominal swelling. The patient may complain of a general increase in girth or of a discrete mass discovered accidentally; alternatively the GP might find the swelling while performing a physical examination.

Differential diagnosis

COMMON
- pregnancy
- irritable bowel syndrome (IBS)
- constipation
- fibroid uterus
- enlarged bladder

OCCASIONAL
- ascites (itself has many causes)
- intestinal obstruction
- ovarian mass (cyst or malignant tumour)
- carcinoma of stomach or colon
- hepatomegaly (various causes)

RARE
- splenomegaly (various causes)
- pancreatic carcinoma
- aortic aneurysm
- massive para-aortic lymphadenopathy
- hydronephrosis, renal cysts and renal malignancy

Ready reckoner

	Pregnancy	IBS	Constipation	Fibroid uterus	Bladder
Size varies	No	Yes	Possible	No	Possible
Amenorrhoea	Yes	No	No	No	No
Poor urinary stream	No	No	No	No	Yes
Diarrhoea	No	Yes	Possible	No	No
Cannot get below	Yes	No	Possible	Yes	Yes

Possible investigations

LIKELY: pregnancy test, ultrasound.

POSSIBLE: urinalysis, FBC, U&E, LFT, CA-125, plain abdomen X-ray.

SMALL PRINT: barium enema and sigmoidoscopy, paracentesis, CT scan.

- Pregnancy test essential in amenorrhoeic women.
- Urinalysis may reveal microscopic haematuria in renal or bladder tumours.
- Abdominal ultrasound is the quickest and most efficient way to define the source of most abdominal swellings or masses. Ultrasound of pelvis/abdomen may also be indicated according to an elevated CA-125 (see below).
- Full blood count (FBC): anaemia likely in malignancy, possible in fibroids with menorrhagia; also will reveal blood dyscrasias.
- Urea and electrolytes (U&E) may be deranged in gross renal disease. Liver function tests (LFTs) may give a clue to alcoholic hepatomegaly or malignancy. Low albumin in ascites.
- CA-125: may be indicated in women, especially those aged 50 or more, to help exclude ovarian cancer.
- Barium enema and sigmoidoscopy: useful to confirm or exclude colonic disease.
- Plain abdominal X-ray: may show constipation or obstruction (in the latter case, likely to be arranged after admission).
- Other tests are likely to be arranged after specialist referral, e.g. paracentesis (to investigate and relieve ascites), CT scanning (to establish nature of mass and its effects on surrounding structures).

TOP TIPS

- Take care in the history to distinguish between intermittent or variable swelling, and progressive swelling. The former will probably not be caused by serious pathology, whereas the latter may well be.
- Pregnancy can catch out the unwary, particularly when dealing with perimenopausal women or teenage girls. Do not accept the claim that 'I can't be pregnant'.
- Some 'swellings' turn out, on examination, to be impalpable or to represent normal

anatomy. The physical examination may have a therapeutic effect. If not, explore the patient's concerns more fully and consider anxiety, depression or other psychological problems if symptoms persist.

Red flags

- ✓ Weight loss in conjunction with abdominal swelling should immediately suggest malignancy.
- ✓ Acute onset of swelling with abdominal pain suggests obstruction, requiring urgent surgical attention.
- ✓ Obesity presents difficulties in examination and can be difficult to distinguish from ascites. If in doubt, arrange an ultrasound.
- ✓ Resonance on percussion does not rule out a solid mass: retroperitoneal masses will push bowel anteriorly and may be apparently tympanic.

NOTES:

ACUTE ABDOMINAL PAIN IN ADULTS

The GP overview

The sudden onset of severe abdominal pain represents a genuine emergency in general practice and is a common out-of-hours call. In the true acute abdomen, the patient is obviously ill, and as the clinical condition may deteriorate rapidly, ensure that you examine the patient as soon as possible.

NOTE: upper and mid-abdominal pain are dealt with here. Lower abdominal pain is dealt with under 'acute pelvic pain' and specifically epigastric-type pain is covered in more detail in the epigastric pain section.

Differential diagnosis

COMMON
- peptic ulcer
- biliary colic
- appendicitis
- gastroenteritis
- renal colic

OCCASIONAL
- cholecystitis (may follow biliary colic, but pain is constant and fever present)
- diverticulitis
- acute or subacute bowel obstruction (adhesions, carcinoma, strangulated hernia, volvulus)
- pyelonephritis
- muscular wall pain
- pancreatitis

RARE
- perforation (e.g. duodenal ulcer (DU), carcinoma) resulting in peritonitis
- hepatitis
- Crohn's and ulcerative colitis
- ischaemic bowel
- dissecting/leaking aneurysm
- diabetic ketoacidosis (DKA) and other occasional medical causes (e.g. myocardial infarction (MI), pneumonia, sickle cell crisis)

Ready reckoner

	Peptic ulcer	Renal colic	Biliary colic	Appendicitis	Gastroenteritis
Colicky pain	No	Yes	Yes	No	Yes
Localised pain	Yes	Yes	Yes	Yes	No
Abdominal tenderness	Yes	No	Possible	Yes	Possible
Fever	No	No	No	Yes	Possible
Diarrhoea	No	No	No	Possible	Yes

Possible investigations

The only test likely to help the GP is urinalysis: this may reveal haematuria (renal colic), evidence of urinary infection, or glycosuria in DKA. In general, the following investigations will be done in hospital after acute admission.

- Full blood count: WCC raised in many causes and confirms acute inflammation or infection.
- U&E essential as abnormalities common with diarrhoea or vomiting. Amylase raised in ischaemic bowel and acute pancreatitis.
- LFT may show raised bilirubin in biliary obstruction, and widespread derangement in hepatitis.
- *Helicobacter pylori* testing: strong association with peptic ulcer disease.
- Upper GI endoscopy: to visualise upper GI tract.
- Plain erect abdominal X-ray invaluable to confirm perforated viscus (air under diaphragm). Supine also necessary if obstruction suspected. Ninety per cent of renal or ureteric stones will be revealed with a plain abdominal X-ray.
- Ultrasound: helpful to confirm gallstones.
- IVU: for ureteric stones.

TOP TIPS

- The aim of assessment is correct disposal rather than an exact diagnosis. Colicky pain may be appropriate to manage at home; constant pain with tenderness is likely to need admission.
- If treating a patient at home, arrange for review as appropriate and ensure that the patient is aware of the symptoms which should prompt urgent reassessment.
- The examination is likely to contribute significantly to making the diagnosis – so take particular care and don't forget the basics such as pulse rate, temperature, bowel sounds and a rectal examination.

☑ Beware 'gastroenteritis' masking or developing into an acute appendicitis. Make arrangements for follow-up and emphasise that constant pain needs urgent review.

☑ Prejudice is easy if the patient has a history of functional problems or irritable bowel. Surgical pathology can happen to anyone, so be objective.

☑ Beware the elderly patient with an irregular pulse: mesenteric infarction causes severe pain but few signs.

☑ Don't forget to examine the hernial orifices, especially if obstruction is a possibility.

NOTES:

ACUTE ABDOMINAL PAIN IN PREGNANCY

The GP overview

A pregnant woman who develops this symptom is very likely to be extremely concerned that there is a threat to her pregnancy. Anxiety levels may therefore be high in the patient and her partner. Acknowledge this emotional distress by an urgent and full assessment. Listed here are causes specific to pregnancy and conditions which may be exacerbated or altered by pregnancy; 'run of the mill' causes (such as gastroenteritis, IBS and dyspepsia) may obviously occur too, but rarely create diagnostic problems and so are not considered in this section.

Differential diagnosis

COMMON
- symphysis pubis and ligament strain
- miscarriage: 20–40% of pregnancies in first trimester
- labour: 6% premature
- placental abruption: 1/80–200 pregnancies
- pyelonephritis (especially around 20 weeks)

OCCASIONAL
- constipation (common cause but only occasionally presents)
- ectopic pregnancy (1/250 pregnancies)
- appendicitis (1/1000 pregnancies)
- red degeneration of fibroid
- torsion/rupture of ovarian cyst or tumour

RARE
- uterine rupture (in UK 1/1500 pregnancies, of which 70% due to Caesarian scar dehiscence)
- uterine torsion (axial rotation >90°): 90% associated with fibroids, adnexal masses and anatomical uterine anomalies
- liver congestion due to pre-eclampsia
- rectus sheath haematoma

Ready reckoner

	S. pubis strain	Miscarriage	Labour	Abruption	Pyelonephritis
Localised tenderness	Yes	No	No	Possible	Yes
Crampy pain	No	Yes	Yes	No	No
Vaginal bleeding	No	Yes	No	Yes	No
Uterine rigidity	No	No	No	Yes	No
Fever, unilateral pain	No	No	No	No	Yes

Possible investigations

These will be dictated by the clinical urgency of the situation. In severe pain, they will be done in secondary care.

LIKELY: urinalysis, MSU.

POSSIBLE: ultrasound, FBC.

SMALL PRINT: laparoscopy.

- ◪ Urinalysis: proteinuria in pre-eclampsia. Blood, pus cells and nitrite in urinary tract infection (UTI); the infecting organism will be confirmed on MSU.
- ◪ FBC: raised WCC in UTI.
- ◪ Imaging ultrasound can be diagnostic in abruption and miscarriage; the presence of an intrauterine pregnancy makes an ectopic very unlikely; ultrasound may also be helpful in detecting a rectus sheath haematoma.
- ◪ Laparoscopy: to confirm ectopic pregnancy.

TOP TIPS

- ◪ Pain on standing and walking, and relieved by rest, with exquisite pubic symphysis tenderness, is 'symphyseal pain' – an often overlooked cause.
- ◪ Allay understandable anxieties as appropriate – particularly regarding the well-being of the foetus or the possibility of premature labour.
- ◪ Do not be too ready to diagnose UTI on the basis of an abnormal urinalysis – contamination in pregnancy is common.

- Distortion of anatomy may alter symptoms and signs: appendicitis is notoriously difficult to diagnose in the second trimester. If in doubt, admit.
- A woman in early pregnancy who experiences unilateral lower abdominal pain followed by light bleeding or blackish discharge has an ectopic until proved otherwise.
- Don't overlook the diagnosis of premature labour. Women with no previous experience of labour pain might not consider this possibility.
- Placental abruption causes severe, continuous pain with a tender, hard uterus. Vaginal bleeding may be minimal. Admit immediately.
- Don't forget pre-eclampsia as a cause of epigastric pain in the third trimester: check the blood pressure (BP) and urine.

NOTES:

CHRONIC/RECURRENT ABDOMINAL PAIN IN ADULTS

The GP overview

This problem may present in any age group. The causes in children are covered in another section. In young to middle-aged adults, the cause is very likely to be benign, but this alters with age: malignancy should always be suspected in the elderly even though other causes are still commoner. A precise diagnosis sometimes remains elusive.

Differential diagnosis

COMMON
- IBS
- recurrent UTI
- chronic peptic ulcer (PU)
- constipation
- diverticular disease

OCCASIONAL
- gallstones
- hydronephrosis
- post-herpetic neuralgia
- inflammatory bowel disease
- ureteric colic
- spinal arthritis
- coeliac disease (commoner than traditionally thought: 1 in 300 adults)

RARE
- mesenteric artery ischaemia (abdominal angina)
- chronic pancreatitis
- subacute obstruction (adhesions, malignancy and diverticulitis)
- functional (psychogenic) abdominal pain
- malignancy
- metabolic causes, e.g. Addison's disease, porphyria, lead poisoning

Ready reckoner

	IBS	UTI	PU	Constipation	Diverticulitis
High abdominal pain	Possible	No	Yes	Possible	Possible
Colicky	Yes	No	No	Yes	Yes
Weight loss	No	Possible	Possible	No	No
Diarrhoea	Yes	No	No	Possible	Yes
Rectal bleeding	No	No	No	Possible	Possible

Possible investigations

LIKELY: urinalysis, FBC, ESR/CRP, MSU, *H. pylori* testing.

POSSIBLE: U&E, LFT, amylase, coeliac screen, CA-125, plain abdominal X-ray, ultrasound, IVU, barium enema, colonoscopy, gastroscopy.

SMALL PRINT: specialised investigations such as mesenteric angiography and further tests for rare medical causes.

- Urinalysis: blood alone with stone; blood, pus cells and nitrite in UTI.
- MSU: to confirm urinary infection and guide treatment.
- FBC and ESR/CRP: may suggest inflammatory bowel disease, PU or malignancy.
- U&E may be deranged in hydronephrosis, renal stones or Addison's disease.
- LFT and amylase: LFT may be abnormal if carcinoma suspected. Amylase may be raised in pancreatitis and bowel ischaemia.
- Coeliac screen: anti-endomysial and anti-gliadin antibodies: suggest coeliac disease if positive.
- CA-125: especially in women aged 50 or more, may help exclude ovarian cancer.
- *H. pylori* testing: strong association with peptic ulcer disease.
- Plain abdominal X-ray: may reveal constipation, subacute obstruction or kidney stones.
- IVU: for renal stones or recurrent UTI.
- Ultrasound: will show hydronephrosis and gallstones. Pelvic/abdominal ultrasound also indicated if CA-125 elevated.
- Barium enema, colonoscopy: for various lower bowel disorders.
- Gastroscopy: may be required to confirm PU and exclude gastric carcinoma.
- Further tests such as angiography (for mesenteric ischaemia) or investigations for rare medical causes may be arranged after specialist referral.

TOP TIPS

- Simply establishing what provokes or relieves the problem can provide helpful pointers: pain occurring after eating suggests gallstones, PU, gastric carcinoma or mesenteric ischaemia; if relieved by defecation, the likely diagnoses are IBS or constipation.
- In an otherwise well patient, the longer the history the less likely there is to be significant underlying disease.

- Avoid repeated investigation if a patient has already been thoroughly assessed in the past – unless the individual becomes unwell or develops new symptoms. Be frank with the patient by explaining about the 'law of diminishing returns' in investigating chronic unexplained abdominal pain.
- Be prepared to make a positive diagnosis of IBS in a fit young patient if the symptoms are classical and basic investigations are negative; explanation and education are the keys to effective management.

- Weight loss in association with recurrent abdominal pain suggests significant pathology.
- Hard enlarged left supraclavicular nodes (Troisier's sign) are pathognomic of gastric carcinoma.
- Beware that constipation itself is often a symptom rather than a diagnosis. Be sure to establish and treat any underlying cause if it doesn't respond to simple treatment.
- IBS is the commonest diagnosis – but consider other possibilities if the pain is always in the same site, wakes the patient at night or is associated with rectal bleeding or weight loss.

NOTES:

CONSTIPATION

The GP overview

Constipation is defined as the infrequent or difficult evacuation of faeces. One study of a large normal working population showed variation in frequency from three times a day to three times a week. The average GP will see about 18 presentations of constipation each year. In most cases, there is a combination of aetiological factors, and serious causes are rare.

Differential diagnosis

COMMON
- diet and lifestyle (inadequate fibre and ignoring the urge to defecate)
- inactivity (especially in the elderly)
- irritable bowel syndrome (IBS)
- painful perianal conditions: fissure, haemorrhoids, abscess, florid warts
- drugs, e.g. opiates, iron, aluminium hydroxide

OCCASIONAL
- poor fluid intake
- acquired megacolon, e.g. chronic laxative abuse, neurological problems, scleroderma
- diverticulosis (with or without stricture)
- hypothyroidism
- carcinoma of rectum or colon

RARE
- pressure from extracolonic pelvic masses
- acute bowel obstruction (various causes)
- hypercalcaemia
- Crohn's disease with stricture
- infants and children: behavioural ('stool holding'), Hirschsprung's disease

Ready reckoner

	Diet and lifestyle	Inactivity	IBS	Perianal conditions	Drugs
Likely in elderly	Yes	Yes	No	Possible	Yes
'Overflow' diarrhoea	Possible	Yes	No	Possible	Possible
Mucus PR	No	No	Possible	Possible	No
Short history	No	No	Possible	Yes	Possible
PR exam very painful	No	No	No	Yes	No

Possible investigations

LIKELY: none; if suspicion of significant underlying bowel pathology, then FBC, barium enema and sigmoidoscopy/colonoscopy (radiology and endoscopy usually arranged in secondary care).

POSSIBLE: urinalysis, thyroid function tests (TFT).

SMALL PRINT: plain abdominal X-ray, serum calcium, ultrasound, CT scan, biopsy.

- Urinalysis: specific gravity high if inadequate fluid intake.
- FBC: may reveal iron deficiency anaemia if underlying carcinoma.
- TFT and serum calcium: will reveal hypothyroidism or hypercalcaemia.
- Plain abdominal X-ray: may reveal megacolon full of faeces; erect and supine views will show obstruction.
- Barium enema, sigmoidoscopy, colonoscopy: may reveal carcinoma or diverticular disease.
- Ultrasound/CT scan: may be helpful if a pelvic mass is present.
- Biopsy: of suspicious lesions or to confirm Hirschsprung's disease.

TOP TIPS

- Clarify what patients mean by constipation: they often use the term inaccurately (e.g. in reference to a perfectly 'normal' bowel habit or to describe another symptom such as tenesmus).
- The longer the history, the less likely there is to be any underlying or remediable cause.
- Check the medication history (including over-the-counter treatment): just about any medication can alter the bowel habit.
- Look at the patient: your immediate impression may give important clues to the underlying diagnosis (e.g. hypothyroidism or weight loss in malignancy).

- Constipation alone in the elderly is rarely caused by sinister pathology – but if it is accompanied by other significant symptoms, such as weight loss, rectal bleeding or mucus, or diarrhoea, carcinoma is likely.
- Beware of attributing abdominal pain to constipation – the true diagnosis might be intestinal obstruction. Visible peristalsis with audible borborygmi is never due to simple constipation.
- Cases of Hirschsprung's disease can present 'late' – consider the diagnosis in a child with chronic constipation, a persistently swollen abdomen and an empty rectum.
- Beware of assuming that known pathology (such as diverticular disease or IBS) in an individual is the cause of constipation. If the patient has presented with constipation, then there may have been a significant change in the pattern or the nature of the symptoms.

NOTES:

DIARRHOEA

The GP overview

Diarrhoea is the passage of abnormally liquid and frequent stools. It is said to be chronic if it lasts more than 2 weeks. It is the fifth-commonest presenting symptom in general practice. Patients will use the term 'diarrhoea' when presenting, but they may just mean frequent stools.

Differential diagnosis

COMMON
- acute infective gastroenteritis, e.g. rotavirus, campylobacter, food poisoning
- antibiotics (and other drug side effects)
- irritable bowel syndrome (IBS)
- diverticulitis
- overflow constipation (especially in the elderly)

OCCASIONAL
- lactose intolerance
- chronic infection: amoebiasis, giardiasis, hookworm
- bowel neoplasia
- inflammatory bowel disease (IBD): ulcerative colitis and Crohn's disease
- excess alcohol
- toddler diarrhoea
- coeliac disease (1 in 300)

RARE
- appendicitis
- laxative misuse
- thyrotoxicosis
- malabsorption, e.g. coeliac disease
- allergy
- ovarian cancer

Ready reckoner

	Gastroenteritis	Antibiotics	IBS	Diverticulitis	Overflow
Vomiting too	Possible	Possible	No	Possible	No
Chronic or recurrent	No	No	Yes	Possible	Yes
Constant severe pain	No	No	No	Yes	No
Marked abdominal tenderness	No	No	No	Yes	No
Blood in stool	Possible	Possible	No	Possible	No

Possible investigations

LIKELY: if persistent, stool specimen, FBC, ESR/CRP, TFT, anti-endomysial and anti-gliadin antibodies, faecal calprotectin.

POSSIBLE: urinalysis, LFT, proctosopy/sigmoidoscopy followed by barium enema, colonoscopy, CA-125.

SMALL PRINT: tests for malabsorption.

- ☑ One stool sample is sufficient in acute diarrhoea of more than a week to look for common infections. Follow-up needed to show clearance of salmonella.
- ☑ Series of three daily stool samples necessary to look for ova, cysts and parasites in chronic diarrhoea.
- ☑ FBC: Hb may be reduced and ESR/CRP elevated in IBD and malignancy; iron deficiency anaemia in neoplasia, coeliac disease; diverticulitis – check ferritin, B_{12} and folate too; WCC raised in IBD and infection.
- ☑ TFT: will reveal thyrotoxicosis.
- ☑ Anti-endomysial and anti-gliadin antibodies: suggest coeliac disease if positive.
- ☑ Faecal calprotectin: helps rule out inflammatory bowel disease.
- ☑ LFT: may suggest secondaries or alcoholism.
- ☑ Urinalysis: specific gravity high in dehydration.
- ☑ Proctoscopy/sigmoidoscopy followed by barium enema or colonoscopy (usually arranged by the specialist): will confirm diagnosis of malignancy, diverticulosis, carcinoma and IBD.
- ☑ CA-125: to help exclude ovarian cancer – especially in women aged 50 or more.
- ☑ Tests for malabsorption: such as stool fat analysis, lactose tolerance test, small intestinal biopsy (all secondary care).

TOP TIPS

- ☑ Clarify what patients mean by diarrhoea – they may be referring simply to a minor change in their normal habit or the frequent passage of normal stools.
- ☑ Giardiasis is much more common than previously thought and may be difficult to isolate in stool specimens. Empirical treatment is justified if the clinical picture is suggestive (recent onset after travel of persistent fatty diarrhoea with anorexia, nausea and bloating).

- IBS rarely causes nocturnal diarrhoea.
- Patients with gastroenteritis should steadily improve after a few days, but may experience symptoms for up to 10 days – warn them of this.
- Do not be caught out by overflow diarrhoea in the elderly. The only way to establish this diagnosis is with a PR.
- Remember to ask about foreign travel and occupation, which have implications for diagnostic possibilities and management.

Red flags

- Weight loss in chronic diarrhoea is highly suggestive of significant pathology.
- In a young and otherwise well person, it is reasonable to make a positive clinical diagnosis of irritable bowel syndrome with minimal investigation – but beware of making this diagnosis for the first time in the middle-aged and elderly. Significant pathology mimicking IBS is likely.
- Carefully assess hydration in infants and the elderly with diarrhoea; if there are signs of dehydration, always admit to hospital.
- Initial telephone consultation is sufficient for most cases of acute diarrhoea, but if in constant (not colicky) abdominal pain, always see and examine to exclude an acute surgical condition.
- Remember that acute diarrhoea in the elderly can precipitate or aggravate renal failure – especially if they are on ACE inhibitors. Stop these drugs for the duration of the illness and ensure adequate hydration.

NOTES:

EPIGASTRIC PAIN

The GP overview

Up to 40% of the adult population suffer this symptom in any 1 year. Only about one in ten seek help from their GP, usually presenting with 'indigestion'. The first step involves sorting out exactly what the patient means by this term. The second is to establish whether it is acute, chronic, or acute-on-chronic. And the third revolves around management, which is often orientated towards a pragmatic, symptomatic approach rather than establishing a precise diagnosis.

Differential diagnosis

COMMON
- non ulcer dyspepsia (NUD)
- gastro-oesophageal reflux disease (GORD)/gastritis
- IBS
- gallstones
- duodenal ulcer/duodenitis

OCCASIONAL
- drug related, e.g. antibiotics, NSAIDs, bisphosphonates
- pancreatitis (acute or chronic)
- muscular
- peritonitis (perforated DU or carcinoma)
- carcinoma of the stomach
- gastric ulcer
- oesophageal spasm
- aerophagy

RARE
- myocardial infarct
- pneumonia
- carcinoma of the pancreas
- ruptured abdominal aortic aneurysm
- gastrointestinal obstruction
- referred from spine
- epigastric hernia

Ready reckoner

	NUD	GORD/gastritis	IBS	Gallstones	DU/duodenitis
Nocturnal pain	Possible	Possible	No	Possible	Yes
Relief with antacids	Possible	Yes	No	No	Possible
Stress related	Possible	Possible	Yes	No	Possible
Radiates to back	No	No	No	Possible	Possible
Vomiting	No	No	No	Possible	Possible

Possible investigations

LIKELY: FBC, *H. pylori* testing.

POSSIBLE: LFT, upper GI endoscopy, ultrasound.

SMALL PRINT: serum amylase, barium swallow or meal, oesophageal manometry/pH studies, cardiac enzymes, ECG, CXR, erect and supine abdominal X-rays.

- FBC: anaemia in underlying malignancy or bleeding from peptic ulcer; WCC raised in cholecystitis and pancreatitis.
- *H. pylori* testing: strong association with peptic ulcer disease; possibly also with other gastrointestinal pathologies.
- LFT: may be abnormal in gallstones or malignancy.
- Upper GI endoscopy: to visualise/biopsy the upper GI tract (in particular, to exclude carcinoma of the stomach).
- Ultrasound: for gallstones; may reveal other pathology such as pancreatic disease.
- Barium swallow or meal: for investigation of the oesophagus, stomach and duodenum in those unwilling to have, or unfit for, endoscopy.
- Serum amylase: elevated in acute pancreatitis.
- Other tests: these are likely to be initiated in secondary care after referral. They include oesophageal manometry/pH studies (if likely oesophageal problem but a normal endoscopy), cardiac enzymes and ECG (possible acute cardiac event), CXR (pneumonia), erect and supine abdominal X-rays (obstruction), CT or MRI scan if a mass is suspected.

TOP TIPS

- The non acute case of 'dyspepsia' in primary care is likely to be managed according to the prevailing guidelines – in which case a precise diagnosis may not be necessary.
- It's important to address underlying concerns. Most patients with epigastric pain do not seek medical help. Those that do usually fear significant disease such as cancer.
- A diagnosis of peptic ulcer still frightens many patients, especially older age groups, as they may be unaware of recent therapeutic advances. Provide adequate explanation and reassurance.

- Don't overlook the medication history, as this may provide a simple solution to the problem.
- A normal endoscopy does not rule out oesophageal problems such as GORD or spasm.

Red flags

- Patients with the following should be referred for endoscopy/other investigations to exclude malignant disease: new onset of symptoms – or significant change in longer term symptoms – in the over-55s with unexplained and persistent dyspepsia; weight loss; dysphagia; GI bleed; vomiting; abdominal mass; anaemia.
- In an obviously unwell patient with weight loss and epigastric pain, do not be 'reassured' by a normal endoscopy. There may well still be significant pathology such as carcinoma of the pancreas.
- In at least 50% of cases, carcinoma of the pancreas presents with epigastric pain rather than the classical painless, progressive jaundice.
- In acute cases, do not overlook referred pain – from heart, lungs or spine.

NOTES:

RECURRENT CHILDHOOD ABDOMINAL PAIN

The GP overview

Recurrent abdominal pain in childhood can be a calling card for a myriad hidden agendas. More than 85 causes have been listed, and as in most areas of general practice, the trick is to sift through the morass of information to find the keys to the diagnosis and open the way to effective management. The underlying cause in the most persistent cases is usually non-organic (90% of those referred to hospital).

Differential diagnosis

COMMON
- recurrent viral illnesses
- anxiety and depression (sometimes known as periodic syndrome or abdominal migraine)
- recurrent UTI
- constipation
- gastritis and GORD

OCCASIONAL
- Crohn's and coeliac disease
- duodenal ulcer (DU)
- irritable bowel syndrome
- diabetes mellitus
- Henoch–Schönlein purpura
- hydronephrosis, renal stones and ureteric reflux
- Meckel's diverticulum

RARE
- parasitic infestation of the gut
- food allergy
- sickle-cell disease
- tuberculosis (TB)
- Hirschsprung's disease
- temporal lobe epilepsy
- pica

Ready reckoner

	Recurrent viral illness	Anxiety/ depression	Recurrent UTI	Constipation	Gastritis/ GORD
School/home stress	No	Yes	No	No	No
Related to eating	No	No	No	Possible	Possible
Diarrhoea	Possible	Possible	No	Possible	No
Fever	Yes	No	Yes	No	No
Abnormal urinalysis	Possible	No	Yes	No	No

Possible investigations

LIKELY: urinalysis, MSU.

POSSIBLE: FBC, blood film, ESR/CRP, anti-endomysial and anti-gliadin antibodies.

SMALL PRINT: plain abdominal X-ray, abdominal ultrasound, further hospital-based investigations (after referral).

- Urinalysis and MSU: urinalysis will reveal evidence of a UTI, which will be confirmed with an MSU for microscopy and culture. Urinalysis will also reveal glucose in diabetes and possible haematuria in Henoch–Schönlein purpura.
- FBC: Hb may be reduced in any chronic disorder; leucocytosis in bacterial infection; eosinophilia in parasitic infestation or genuine food allergy. Blood film may show sickling. Raised ESR/CRP suggests organic disease.
- Anti-endomysial and anti-gliadin antibodies: a positive result suggests coeliac disease.
- Ultrasound: non-invasive first line investigation of renal tract. Other investigation for confirmed UTI will be arranged by the paediatrician.
- Further hospital-based investigations: if there is a high suspicion of organic disease, e.g. endoscopy for DU, barium meal and follow-through for Crohn's disease.

TOP TIPS

- The majority of children with recurrent abdominal pain will not have organic pathology – take the problem seriously and assess carefully, but avoid reinforcing worries with unnecessary investigation or referral.
- Explore the parents' concerns – a child's anxiety may be fed by parents unnecessarily worrying about sinister and unlikely diagnoses.
- Talk to children alone – this may reveal relevant problems at home or school which they would not have been able to admit in front of parents.
- If recurrent UTI is a possibility, provide the parents with the necessary bottle and lab form so that an MSU can be taken during the next episode of pain.

- Organic disease is suggested by pain distant from the umbilicus which wakes the child and which is associated with loss of appetite or weight, or a change in bowel habit.
- Beware the unlikely event of an acute cause for the pain supervening, e.g. appendicitis, torsion of the testis – ensure that parents know that a different, acute pain should not be dismissed as 'the same old problem', but should be presented urgently.
- Children proven to have a UTI should be managed according to NICE guidelines.
- Avoid colluding in parental somatisation and overlooking the existence of family dysfunction or other causes of unhappiness.
- Don't forget the rare possibility of sickling in the appropriate ethnic groups.

NOTES:

VOMITING

The GP overview

Vomiting is one of the commonest reasons for an out-of-hours call – especially for children. While most cases are self-limiting and benign, the possible causes are numerous and the symptoms can herald serious pathology. Careful assessment is required, together with a willingness to review and admit if the diagnosis remains unclear.

Differential diagnosis

COMMON
- gastroenteritis
- acute viral labyrinthitis (and some other causes of acute vertigo)
- upper respiratory tract infection (URTI) (in children, especially with marked coughing)
- pregnancy
- appendicitis and other causes of the acute abdomen

OCCASIONAL
- hyper- and hypoglycaemia
- intestinal obstruction
- pyelonephritis
- ureteric calculus
- migraine
- medication (e.g. antibiotics and cytotoxics)

RARE
- gastroduodenal disease (e.g. pyloric stricture or stenosis, DU, carcinoma)
- meningitis
- cerebral haemorrhage
- bulimia nervosa
- severe constipation
- raised intracranial pressure (e.g. tumour)
- renal failure
- acute glaucoma

Ready reckoner

	Gastroenteritis	Labyrinthitis	URTI (child)	Pregnancy	Acute abdomen
Mainly mornings	No	No	No	Yes	No
With diarrhoea	Yes	No	Possible	No	Possible
Nystagmus	No	Yes	No	No	No
Bowel sounds increased?	Yes	No	No	No	Possible
Tender abdomen?	Possible	No	Possible	No	Yes

Possible investigations

LIKELY: none.

POSSIBLE: urinalysis, MSU, pregnancy test, blood glucose, FBC, U&E.

SMALL PRINT: lumbar puncture, abdominal X-rays, IVU, OGD, CT scan.

◪ Urinalysis: high specific gravity suggests dehydration; glucose and ketones indicate hyperglycaemia; blood, white cells and protein, with or without nitrites, suggest UTI (confirm with MSU); blood alone might indicate a renal stone.

◪ Pregnancy test: to confirm or reveal pregnancy.

◪ Blood glucose: will confirm hypo- or hyperglycaemia.

◪ U&E: may be deranged by vomiting; may also reveal underlying renal failure.

◪ FBC: raised WCC suggests underlying infection or inflammation. Haemoglobin (Hb) may be reduced in malignancy.

◪ Lumbar puncture, IVU, abdominal X-rays, OGD and CT scans: required in a few cases depending on the clinical picture and invariably arranged by the relevant specialist.

TOP TIPS

◪ Vomiting in children tends to be presented early, when it may be difficult to give a definite diagnosis. Be honest about this and make sure that parents know to call you again if the symptom doesn't settle or other 'alarm' symptoms develop – or arrange a definite time for follow-up.

◪ Remember to look for both the cause (i.e. the aetiology) and the effect (i.e. possible dehydration) – especially in the very young and the very old, when the history may be difficult to obtain and the effects of fluid loss more marked.

◪ Check to see if the patient is on any medication. This may be causing the vomiting, or it may have serious implications for management (e.g. steroids).

◪ Don't forget pregnancy as a cause – the patient may be 'ignoring' the possibility.

Red flags

◪ Unless the diagnosis is obviously migraine, beware the patient with vomiting and a headache – think of meningitis, subarachnoid haemorrhage or raised intracranial pressure.

◪ Do not treat empirically with anti-emetics – these may mask the true diagnosis or cause diagnostic confusion via side effects.

◪ Have a low threshold for admitting diabetics. Whatever the cause of the vomiting, their diabetes is liable to become uncontrolled.

◪ Look for acid dental erosion as a clue to bulimia in recurrent vomiting.

◪ Gastroenteritis should cause increased bowel sounds. In the patient with abdominal pain and vomiting, if bowel sounds are absent or scanty, the diagnosis is likely to be an acute abdomen.

NOTES:

VOMITING BLOOD

The GP overview

This presentation may vary from a few red streaks in gastric fluid to copious quantities of bright red blood. Blood static in the stomach for a few hours will change to look dark and granular, like coffee grounds. Always do a full urgent assessment, and be prepared for the sudden need for resuscitation.

Differential diagnosis

COMMON
- peptic ulcer (PU)/acute gastritis
- Mallory–Weiss (M–W) tear
- oesophageal varices (cirrhosis, usually alcoholic)
- malignancy: oesophagus or stomach
- GORD

OCCASIONAL
- swallowed blood (nose bleeds obvious, haemoptysis less so)
- foreign body or mediastinal tumour perforating oesophagus and aorta (including aneurysm)
- haemobilia (blood in bile)
- ingested poisons: corrosive acid and alkali, arsenic
- blood dyscrasias (e.g. thrombocytopenia, leukaemia, haemophilia, aplastic anaemia)

RARE
- ruptured oesophagus (acute vomiting or trauma)
- spurious: deliberate swallowing and vomiting of blood (Munchausen's syndrome)
- gallstone perforation of duodenum
- scurvy
- polyarteritis nodosa, systemic lupus erythematosus (SLE)

Ready reckoner

	PU	M–W tear	Varices	Cancer	Oesophagitis
History of weight loss	Possible	No	Possible	Yes	No
Preceded by vomiting	Possible	Yes	No	No	No
Preceded by melaena	Possible	No	Possible	Possible	Possible
Severe pain	Yes	Possible	No	Possible	Yes
Signs of shock likely	Yes	No	Yes	Possible	No

Possible investigations

These will be done acutely in hospital, or in general practice after an episode of haematemesis when urgent admission is not indicated.

- ◪ FBC: essential for assessment of the degree of blood loss. A normal Hb does not exclude a serious bleed as haemodilution may take several hours. Will also reveal blood dyscrasias.
- ◪ Upper gastrointestinal (GI) endoscopy is the gold standard for finding the cause of the bleed and biopsy of suspicious lesions.
- ◪ *Helicobacter* testing: in the presence of peptic ulceration.
- ◪ LFT and γGT to assess liver function. Alcohol is a significant contributory factor in many cases.
- ◪ Plain erect abdominal X-ray (in hospital) useful to look for signs of viscus perforation (air under diaphragm) and, rarely, an ectopic gallstone.

TOP TIPS

- ◪ Take a careful history – patients often confuse vomiting up and coughing up blood.
- ◪ If about to visit, ask the patient not to dispose of the evidence – viewing the vomit is worth a thousand words of history.
- ◪ Don't forget the relevance of the patient's drug history: non-steroidal anti-inflammatory drugs (NSAIDs), steroids and warfarin may all be associated with acute gastric erosions.

- Tachycardia may be the only physical sign of a significant GI bleed.
- In all acute cases, admit unless the patient is perfectly well and the cause obvious and insignificant (e.g. swallowed blood or very minor Mallory–Weiss tear).
- The patient may not realise the significance of coffee-ground vomit or melaena – enquire specifically about these symptoms.
- Troisier's sign (enlargement of the left supraclavicular node) strongly suggests malignancy.
- Oesophageal varices account for only 5% of cases, but 80% of mortality. Call for an ambulance immediately and secure intravenous (IV) access if possible.

NOTES:

ANORECTAL

Anal itching

Anal swelling

Anorectal pain

Rectal bleeding

Rectal discharge

ANAL ITCHING

The GP overview

Straight out of the list of 'Embarrassing things to see your GP about', this is a presentation that patients love to hate. From a GP perspective, it's one that is generally straightforward to deal with, and effective treatment can usually be offered immediately, much to the patient's relief.

Differential diagnosis

COMMON
- fungal infection – tinea, thrush
- threadworms
- haemorrhoids
- perianal skin tags
- anal fissure

OCCASIONAL
- poor hygiene
- recurrent or chronic diarrhoea
- perianal warts
- streptococcal perianal infection in children
- trauma from sexual practices – anal intercourse and foreign body insertion
- faecal incontinence, including liquid faecal seepage round impacted scybala
- psoriasis
- secondary to underlying diabetes
- anorectal carcinoma
- chemical irritation: defaecation after a very spicy meal (commonly experienced, rarely presented in practice), bubble baths, soaps, sexual lubricants

RARE
- irritation from perineal decorative body piercing (the 'Guiche')
- lichen sclerosus et atrophicus (affects 1 in 100 women, 3 in 10 of these have anal symptoms)
- Crohn's disease (anal/perianal fistula)
- rectovaginal fistula
- rectal prolapse
- any other cause of rectal discharge or anal swellings – see appropriate chapters
- any serious cause of generalised pruritus – see chapter on anal itching. Rare here because pruritus ani is unlikely to be a presenting complaint
- STDs, e.g. syphilis, gonorrhoea, chlamydia

Ready reckoner

	Fungal infection	Threadworms	Haemorrhoids	Skin tags	Fissure
Rectal bleeding	No	Possible	Possible	No	Yes
Markedly worse at night	Possible	Yes	Possible	Possible	No
Complains of lump	No	No	Possible	Possible	No
Rectal discharge	No	No	Possible	No	Possible
Painful defaecation	No	No	Possible	No	Yes

Possible investigations

LIKELY: none.

POSSIBLE: skin swab, FBC, ESR, fasting glucose or HbA1c, proctoscopy.

SMALL PRINT: none.

- In general, unless there are obvious pointers to other more serious disease, investigations would usually only follow after failure of empirical treatment.
- Skin swab for bacteriology may help identify local infection.
- FBC, ESR: may be helpful if Crohn's disease is suspected, but only as an adjunct to referral as the appropriate management.
- Fasting glucose or HbA1c is essential in recurrent or prolonged cases to exclude diabetes.
- Proctoscopy is quick to do in general practice and can yield valuable information if there is an underlying rectal cause.

TOP TIPS

- Most patients will have attempted self-treatment before presenting in the surgery. This may not always have been appropriate, and could have made the problem worse.
- Unless you are absolutely sure of an obvious cause, it is wise to perform a digital rectal examination to look for rectal causes.
- Perianal warts imply a sexually transmitted disease contact. Refer to GUM clinic for contact tracing and treatment.
- Anal itching is often associated with soreness. If it precludes a rectal examination but there is no obvious primary anal cause for itching, treat symptomatically and bring the patient back to complete the assessment when more comfortable to do so. The patient is unlikely to want to return for this without understanding a clear explanation of why it is necessary.

- Four per cent of women with lichen sclerosus et atrophicus go on to develop vulval cancer. Refer if the vulva is affected, or if treatment fails.
- Refer any suspicious anal lesion for biopsy.
- Be confident to ask about recent sexual encounters and sexual practices if possibly relevant. Sexual history may be important.

NOTES:

ANAL SWELLING

The GP overview

Because of embarrassment on the part of the patient, this may well present as a 'while I'm here' symptom. The temptation to make a diagnosis without examination should be resisted – some of the causes (such as perianal abscesses) require urgent attention and others may, rarely, provide something of a surprise (e.g. fistulae, carcinoma).

Differential diagnosis

COMMON
- prolapsed pile
- perianal haematoma
- skin tags
- perianal abscess
- rectal prolapse

OCCASIONAL
- warts
- sebaceous cyst
- sentinel pile
- infected pilonidal sinus

RARE
- hidradenitis
- anal fistula
- carcinoma

Ready reckoner

	Prolapsed pile	Perianal haematoma	Skin tags	Perianal abscess	Rectal prolapse
Painful	Possible	Yes	No	Yes	No
Intermittent	Possible	No	No	No	Possible
Constipated	Possible	Possible	No	Possible	Possible
Long history	Possible	No	Yes	No	Possible
Rectal bleeding	Possible	Possible	No	Possible	No

Possible investigations

In most cases, investigation will be unnecessary. The only exceptions are warts (in which case referral to the local GUM clinic may be required to screen for sexually transmitted disease) and possible carcinoma (in which case biopsy will be performed in secondary care). Also, any suspicion of Crohn's disease causing perianal disease would be investigated in hospital in the usual way.

TOP TIPS

☑ This is one of those situations in which a brief history can be taken while the patient is undressing, or during the examination. Atypically for primary care, it's the examination, rather than the history, which usually provides the definitive diagnosis.

☑ If a discharge, as well as a lump, is mentioned by the patient, then abscesses, warts, prolapses and fistulae top the list of differentials.

☑ The patient with an anal swelling who has obvious difficulty walking into the consulting room has either an abscess, a large perianal haematoma or strangulated prolapsed piles.

Red flags

☑ Recurrent or multiple fistulae suggest Crohn's disease.

☑ If a prolapsed pile is very swollen and painful, it is probably strangulated, and so requires urgent surgical attention.

☑ A persistent, ulcerating anal swelling, especially in the middle-aged or elderly, requires urgent biopsy to exclude carcinoma.

NOTES:

ANORECTAL PAIN

The GP overview

This is usually severe and distressing. Because of reflex sphincteric spasm, constipation very often follows and increases the pain and suffering further. Adequate examination is also difficult for the same reason; fortunately if a PR exam is too difficult, a visual inspection can often yield the diagnosis.

Differential diagnosis

COMMON
- anal fissure
- thrombosed haemorrhoids/perianal haematoma
- perianal abscess
- proctalgia fugax (PF)
- anorectal malignancy

OCCASIONAL
- levator ani syndrome
- Crohn's disease
- coccydynia
- descending perineum syndrome
- prostatitis
- ovarian cyst or tumour
- solitary rectal ulcer syndrome

RARE
- anal tuberculosis
- cauda equina lesion
- endometriosis
- trauma
- presacral tumours

Ready reckoner

	Anal fissure	Haematoma	Abscess	PF	Malignancy
Began while defecating	Yes	No	No	Possible	No
Visible anal swelling	No	Yes	Possible	No	Possible
Pain intermittent	Possible	No	No	Yes	No
Rectal bleeding	Yes	Possible	Possible	No	Yes
PR exam excruciating	Yes	Yes	Yes	Possible	Possible

Possible investigations

LIKELY: none.

POSSIBLE: FBC, ESR/CRP, proctoscopy, faecal calprotectin.

SMALL PRINT: urinalysis, ultrasound, barium enema, other imaging.

- FBC/ESR/CRP: WCC may be raised in abscess and Crohn's disease. ESR/CRP raised in these and carcinoma.
- Proctoscopy valuable if pain allows (specialist might also take biopsy).
- Faecal calprotectin: may help in diagnosing Crohn's disease.
- Urinalysis: pus cells and blood may be present in prostatitis or invasive bladder tumour.
- Ultrasound of pelvis if pelvic examination reveals a mass. Barium enema may be necessary to assess possible bowel involvement. In obscure cases, specialists may request other forms of imaging.

TOP TIPS

- If the patient uses dramatic language (e.g. red-hot poker) to describe fleeting pain, is otherwise well and there are no obvious abnormalities on examination, the diagnosis is likely to be proctalgia fugax.
- Examine the patient – the cause is usually a thrombosed pile, anal fissure or an abscess, and these can usually be diagnosed by simple inspection.
- Provide symptomatic relief but remember to deal with any underlying causes – especially constipation.
- Don't forget to ask about thirst and urinary frequency: recurrent abscesses may be the first presentation of diabetes.

- Preceding weight loss and/or change in bowel habit should prompt a full urgent assessment with carcinoma and inflammatory bowel disease in mind.
- Some perianal abscesses do not result in external swelling. If PR exam is prohibitively painful, consider this possibility – especially if the patient is febrile.
- In florid or recurrent perianal problems, think of Crohn's disease as a possible cause.
- Remember rarer causes in intractable, constant pain in a patient with no obvious signs on PR.

NOTES:

RECTAL BLEEDING

The GP overview

This is a very common presenting complaint and creates a lot of anxiety in the patient. By far the likeliest causes are haemorrhoids or a fissure, but more sinister pathologies should be considered according to the clinical picture. In children, constipation causing a fissure is the most frequent cause.

Differential diagnosis

COMMON
- haemorrhoids
- anal fissure
- gastroenteritis
- rectal carcinoma
- diverticular disease

OCCASIONAL
- villous adenoma
- trauma (especially non-accidental injury (NAI) if in children)
- anticoagulant therapy
- inflammatory bowel disease
- colonic carcinoma

RARE
- blood clotting disorders (including anticoagulants)
- bowel ischaemia
- angiodysplasia
- intussusception
- Meckel's diverticulum (in children)

Ready reckoner

	Piles	Fissure	Gastroenteritis	Cancer of rectum	Diverticulosis
Blood and stool mixed	No	No	Yes	No	Possible
Abdominal pain	No	No	Yes	No	Possible
Diarrhoea	No	No	Yes	No	Yes
Mass felt PR	Possible	No	No	Yes	Possible
Sentinel anal skin tag	No	Yes	No	No	No

Possible investigations

LIKELY: proctoscopy.

POSSIBLE: FBC, ESR/CRP, LFTs, bone biochemistry, U&E, stool for microbiology and faecal calprotectin, sigmoidoscopy, colonoscopy, barium enema.

SMALL PRINT: clotting screen.

- FBC: check for anaemia from acute or chronic bleeding; low platelets may cause or aggravate bleeding.
- ESR/CRP raised in active inflammatory bowel disease and malignancy.
- If malignancy is suspected, LFT, U&E and bone biochemistry are useful early on as a baseline.
- Clotting screen: if clotting disorder a possibility; INR if on warfarin.
- Stool specimen: helpful in the presence of diarrhoea. May show evidence of infective cause (especially *Campylobacter*) or white cells in inflammatory bowel disease. Faecal calprotectin may be useful in diagnosing IBD.
- Proctoscopy: helpful in primary care in visualising haemorrhoids and proctitis to confirm a clinical diagnosis.
- Sigmoidoscopy or colonoscopy are the most helpful investigations if significant pathology is suspected, and allow biopsy of suspicious lesions.
- Barium enema good for revealing strictures related to the underlying pathology, but if diverticulosis present, may not rule out coexistent neoplasia.

TOP TIPS

- Eighty per cent of rectal tumours are within fingertip range. Always do a PR examination unless, in a child or young adult, the diagnosis is manifestly obvious from the history.
- If blood is on the toilet paper and surface of the motions, the cause is likely to be palpable PR or visible on proctoscopy; if mixed in with the motions, referral for further investigation will be required to make a definite diagnosis.
- In young adults, the diagnosis is usually clear from the history and is likely to be haemorrhoids or a fissure. In such cases, if and when you refer, to allay anxiety, emphasise that this is for treatment rather than investigation.

- The presence of diarrhoea with rectal bleeding in young or middle-aged adults suggests gastroenteritis (especially *Campylobacter*) or colitis.

- Change of bowel habit and weight loss with rectal bleeding are ominous symptoms which should prompt urgent referral.
- If a child is presented with rectal bleeding without any clear cause, consider NAI.
- The presence of haemorrhoids does not necessarily clinch the diagnosis – another lesion may be present, especially in the elderly.
- A brisk, painless haemorrhage in an elderly patient is likely to be caused by diverticular disease. Significant amounts of blood can be lost, so assess urgently with a view to admission.

NOTES:

RECTAL DISCHARGE

![line]

The GP overview

This unpleasant symptom causes considerable embarrassment and inconvenience. The presenting complaint may well be itching rather than a history of discharge or dampness. The most common causes are benign, but serious pathology is sufficiently likely to warrant thorough examination.

![line]

Differential diagnosis

COMMON
- haemorrhoids
- anal fissure
- rectal prolapse
- proctitis
- perianal warts

OCCASIONAL
- rectal carcinoma
- IBS
- anal/perianal fistula (may be associated with Crohn's disease)
- villous adenoma
- poor anal hygiene
- solitary rectal ulcer syndrome

RARE
- anal tuberculosis
- anal carcinoma
- STD, e.g. syphilis, gonorrhoea, chlamydia
- AIDS

Ready reckoner

	Piles	Fissure	Prolapse	Proctitis	Warts
Purulent	No	Possible	No	Possible	No
Mucus	Yes	Possible	Yes	Yes	No
Bloodstained	Possible	Yes	Possible	Possible	Possible
Painful PR exam	Possible	Yes	No	Yes	Possible
Associated diarrhoea	No	No	Possible	Yes	No

Possible investigations

LIKELY: swab if purulent.

POSSIBLE: FBC, ESR/CRP, U&E and direct visualisation techniques (see below).

SMALL PRINT: STD screen.

- ◩ Anorectal swab for bacteriology if pus and local inflammation is present.
- ◩ FBC/ESR/CRP: WCC and ESR/CRP raised in inflammatory bowel disease.
- ◩ U&E: profuse mucus discharge from a villous adenoma can cause hypokalaemia.
- ◩ Proctoscopy easily done in practice and guides management and referral.
- ◩ Sigmoidoscopy allows definitive examination and biopsy of suspicious lesions or inflammation.
- ◩ STD screen – if STD suspected.

TOP TIPS

- ◩ This symptom is likely to be associated with embarrassment. A clinical examination is important – so help the patient overcome any reticence with a sympathetic approach.
- ◩ Normal secretions from the anus should not be discounted – from perianal sweat glands and the anal glands themselves. This can sometimes cause a significant problem, particularly in the obese and those with poor anal hygiene.
- ◩ In women, the source of the discharge may be unclear. Speculum examination and protoscopy may be required to resolve any doubt.

■ Sexual history may be important. Don't be coy in asking about recent sexual encounters and sexual practices if relevant.

■ Rectal discharge in the elderly suggests carcinoma unless proved otherwise.

■ A history of diarrhoea and abdominal pain suggests bowel pathology. Ulcerative colitis or Crohn's disease is most likely in this context.

■ Any ulcerating lesion in the perianal area other than an obvious haemorrhoid should prompt referral for biopsy.

NOTES:

BREAST

Breast enlargement in men

Breast lumps in women

Breast pain

Nipple discharge

BREAST ENLARGEMENT IN MEN

The GP overview

Swelling of the breast tissue in a male is an embarrassing symptom, often presented behind the facade of a 'calling card'. The following differential diagnosis does not include other causes of breast swelling, which are referred to in the Top tips at the end of this section. In true breast swelling, glandular tissue is palpable behind the areola and is usually bilateral.

Differential diagnosis

COMMON
- ☑ puberty
- ☑ drugs (spironolactone, cimetidine, digoxin, cyproterone, finasteride, marijuana)
- ☑ chronic liver disease (especially alcohol)
- ☑ lung carcinoma
- ☑ hyperthyroidism

OCCASIONAL
- ☑ hypothyroidism
- ☑ hyperprolactinaemia
- ☑ haemodialysis and chronic renal failure
- ☑ testicular carcinoma
- ☑ adrenal carcinoma
- ☑ cryptorchidism and other causes of hypogonadism

RARE
- ☑ Klinefelter's syndrome
- ☑ true hermaphroditism and male pseudohermaphroditism
- ☑ acromegaly
- ☑ McCune–Albright syndrome
- ☑ hypernephroma
- ☑ carcinoma

Ready reckoner

	Puberty	Drugs	Liver disease	Lung cancer	Hyperthyroidism
Often unilateral	Yes	No	No	No	No
Cough	No	No	No	Yes	No
Weight loss	No	No	Possible	Yes	Yes
Generally unwell	No	Possible	Yes	Yes	Yes
Other physical signs	No	Possible	Yes	Yes	Possible

Possible investigations

LIKELY (except for obvious pubertal cause): FBC, U&E, LFT, TFT.

POSSIBLE: testosterone, CXR, tests of pituitary function.

SMALL PRINT: tumour markers, chromosome analysis, CT scan, biopsy.

- FBC: many chronic systemic illnesses can cause gynaecomastia. There may be an associated normochromic, normocytic anaemia. MCV may be raised in hypothyroidism and chronic liver disease.
- U&E and LFT: will reveal chronic renal and liver disease.
- TFT: to diagnose thyroid abnormality.
- Testosterone: reduced in hypogonadism and chronic illness including liver disease.
- CXR: if lung carcinoma a possibility.
- Tests of pituitary function (e.g. FSH, LH, prolactin and other more complex, hospital-based tests): to check for pituitary hormone abnormalities.
- Tumour markers (usually hospital-based): AFP and HCG act as tumour markers for testicular carcinoma.
- Chromosome analysis: for Klinefelter's syndrome.
- CT scan (secondary care): may be necessary for testicular tumour staging and diagnosis of adrenal and renal tumours.
- Biopsy: if carcinoma suspected.

TOP TIPS

- Many male breast swellings are not true breast enlargement: possibilities include simple obesity, abscess, sebaceous cyst and lipoma.
- Pubertal boys will be very self-conscious about gynaecomastia. Reassure them that the problem is common and will resolve, and that they are not changing sex.
- Iatrogenic causes are common – check the drug history (including over-the-counter and illicit drugs).

- In a pubertal boy with a 'normal' and a 'small' testis, the 'normal' one may conceal a tumour. Check with an ultrasound if in doubt.
- Apparent unilateral gynaecomastia in an adult male may be due to breast carcinoma – refer urgently if there is a hard mass, you cannot feel glandular tissue behind the areola, or you're in any doubt.
- Gynaecomastia with a headache and visual disturbance may be caused by a pituitary tumour. Refer urgently.
- Clubbing of the fingers in a smoker with gynaecomastia is virtually pathognomic of bronchial carcinoma. Investigate urgently.

NOTES:

BREAST LUMPS IN WOMEN

The GP overview

The discovery of a lump in a woman's breast will usually create a lot of anxiety. She will probably have found it herself and with the high public awareness of breast cancer, will want reassurance or rapid action. A careful examination of both breasts and associated lymph nodes is mandatory.

Differential diagnosis

COMMON
- carcinoma
- cyst
- abscess
- fibroadenoma
- fibrous dysplasia

OCCASIONAL
- duct ectasia
- fat necrosis
- lipoma
- Paget's disease of the nipple
- galactocoele
- multiple cysts

RARE
- tuberculosis
- sarcoma
- lymphoma
- phyllodes tumour (benign)
- Mondor's disease (thrombophlebitis)

Ready reckoner

	Cancer	Cyst	Abscess	Fibroadenoma	Fibrous dysplasia
Changes with periods	No	Possible	No	No	Yes
Discharge	Possible	No	Possible	No	Possible
Painful	Possible	Possible	Yes	No	Possible
Bilateral	Possible	Possible	No	Possible	Yes
Highly mobile	Possible	No	No	Yes	No

Possible investigations

There are few investigations worth doing in general practice other than attempted aspiration of a suspected cyst.

Specialist investigation may include aspiration, mammography, ultrasound (for example, to distinguish a solid from a cystic lump), biopsy and, when appropriate, cancer staging.

TOP TIPS

- If the lump feels cystic, consider aspiration – instant resolution of the problem will result in a very grateful patient. But warn the patient that unsuccessful aspiration, while requiring referral, does not necessarily imply a sinister diagnosis – some cysts can be very difficult to aspirate.
- Check the breast again a couple of weeks after aspiration. As long as the lump has completely resolved and the aspirate was not bloodstained, no further action is required.
- It is quite common for women to think they can feel a lump while the doctor has difficulty in detecting a discrete lesion. Re-examine after the patient's next period – but then make a firm management decision. If in doubt, refer rather than delay further as the woman will understandably be very anxious.
- In the very elderly, breast carcinoma may run a relatively benign course, responding very well to tamoxifen alone. In certain cases it might be worth discussing the situation with your local specialist, as GP treatment will provoke far less anxiety.

- Skin dimpling, local flattening of the breast and nipple alteration indicate cancer until proved otherwise.
- Even if the diagnosis is likely to be a fibroadenoma – as in a young woman with a highly mobile lump – refer, as unpleasant surprises do occur.
- In a post-menopausal woman, the diagnosis is almost certain to be carcinoma. Refer urgently.
- A mass appearing after trauma may be fat necrosis – but recheck after a few weeks and refer if not resolved.

NOTES:

BREAST PAIN

The GP overview

Breast pain have a variety of innocent causes: the commonest are puberty and pregnancy. It can be a troublesome recurrent problem for women with cyclical mastalgia. Cancer is very likely to be a major concern: this is an uncommon cause and pain is an unfortunately late sign of the disease.

Differential diagnosis

COMMON
- pregnancy
- cyclical mastalgia
- cracked or inflamed nipple
- breast abscess
- mastitis

OCCASIONAL
- carcinoma
- onset of puberty
- lactation and/or galactocoele
- simple cyst
- trauma

RARE
- chondritis of costal cartilage
- angina
- cervical spondylosis
- herpes zoster
- Mondor's disease (thrombophlebitis of chest wall or breast veins – rare: 0.5–0.9%)
- tuberculosis

Ready reckoner

	Pregnancy	Cyclical mastalgia	Inflamed nipple	Abscess	Mastitis
Bilateral	Yes	Yes	No	No	No
Fever	No	No	No	Yes	Yes
Discrete mass	No	No	No	Yes	No
Local erythema	No	No	Yes	Possible	Yes
Diffuse nodularity	Possible	Yes	No	No	No

Possible investigations

LIKELY: none.

POSSIBLE: pregnancy test, fine needle aspiration, mammography.

SMALL PRINT: swab of any nipple discharge, other investigations if non-breast causes suspected.

- Pregnancy test worthwhile in bilateral pain if a period has been missed.
- Fine needle aspiration of a tense cyst may yield fluid for cytology and relieve the pain. If only blood is obtained, refer urgently.
- Mammography may help if pain is accompanied by a mass or ill-defined nodularity but this would normally be performed in secondary care after referral.
- If the aetiology is infective and the nipple is discharging, a swab may help guide treatment.
- Other investigations: if a non-breast cause is suspected, other tests may be required according to the pattern of the symptoms, e.g. stress test (angina) or cervical spine X-ray (cervical spondylosis).

TOP TIPS

- Offer to examine the breasts even if you are sure from the history that there is no significant pathology – many women fear breast cancer and will find your reassurance hard to accept if they feel they haven't been taken seriously.
- Don't reflexly prescribe in cyclical mastalgia; the patient's agenda is often to exclude serious disease rather than seek drug therapy.
- Remember pregnancy as a cause – the patient will not always volunteer this as a possibility, even if she has just missed a period.
- Unilateral breast pain with no other local signs may be an early symptom of shingles. Check the back in the T4/5 dermatomes for a rash.

- 'Chest pain' may be a euphemism used by a (frequently older) woman in denial. Don't miss advanced tumour through not examining the breasts.
- Cancer rarely presents with breast pain but consider this possibility in a woman complaining of constant 'pricking' breast pain.
- A lactating woman with unilateral breast pain and flu-type symptoms is probably developing mastitis – treat early to avoid the development of an abscess.
- If the pain is related to exertion in a late middle-aged or elderly woman, consider angina as a possibility.

NOTES:

NIPPLE DISCHARGE

The GP overview

Nipple discharge has a number of disparate causes, from the first outward sign of a previously unrecognised pregnancy, to a late sign of an advanced carcinoma. It can cause embarrassment and concern in equally large amounts. Compared with breast pain and lumps, it is a relatively rare presenting symptom. Take it seriously and assess carefully – investigation will often be needed.

Differential diagnosis

COMMON
- pregnancy
- duct papilloma
- duct ectasia
- acute mastitis/breast abscess
- areolar abscess (infected gland of Montgomery)

OCCASIONAL
- oral contraceptives
- intraduct carcinoma
- neonatal and peripubertal galactorrhoea (also post-lactation)
- hyperprolactinaemia (drugs, prolactinoma, hypothyroidism)
- duct epithelial proliferation
- galactocoele

RARE
- periductal (plasma cell) mastitis
- mechanical stimulation
- invasive carcinoma
- tuberculous abscess
- mamillary duct fistula
- Paget's disease of nipple
- comedo mastitis

Ready reckoner

	Pregnancy	Papilloma	Ectasia	Mastitis	Areolar abscess
Bloodstained	No	Yes	Possible	Possible	Possible
Multicoloured/cheesy	No	No	Yes	No	No
Purulent	No	No	No	Yes	Yes
Hot tender segment	No	No	No	Yes	Yes
Bilateral	Yes	No	Possible	No	No

Possible investigations

LIKELY: none (referral for biopsy or mammogram in suspicious cases).

OCCASIONAL: pregnancy test, prolactin level, TFT.

SMALL PRINT: swab of purulent discharge.

- Pregnancy test if pregnancy suspected.
- Swab purulent discharge: may help guide antibiotic therapy.
- Prolactin level and TFT: to check for hyperprolactinaemia or hypothyroidism in galactorrhoea.
- Excision biopsy will be performed if a suspicious lump is palpable. In cases of doubt, mammography may help; surgical exploration may also be undertaken if pressure on an area of one breast consistently elicits discharge.

TOP TIPS

- Women presenting with breast discharge are likely to be afraid there may be an underlying cancer. To 'reassure' properly, make sure you address this anxiety.
- If the discharge is bilateral, then serious breast disease is highly unlikely.
- In a woman of child-bearing age with bilateral serous discharge, enquire specifically about pregnancy: this possibility may be deliberately concealed or genuinely overlooked by the patient.
- If a pre-menopausal woman is amenorrhoeic with bilateral discharge and pregnancy has been excluded, remember the possibility of hyperprolactinaemia.

☑ Women with new breast discharge over the age of 50 (unless there is an obvious benign cause), and all women with bloody discharge, should be referred to exclude serious pathology.

☑ If a lump is palpable, or pressure on a certain area of the breast consistently produces the discharge, refer for probable excision biopsy.

☑ Bright red blood from one orifice suggests duct papilloma or carcinoma.

☑ Nipple discharge in a male is always abnormal, except occasionally in pubertal boys. Investigate or refer as appropriate.

NOTES:

CEREBRAL

Acute confusion

Dizziness

Hallucinations

Headache

Insomnia

Loss of libido

Memory loss

Vertigo

ACUTE CONFUSION

The GP overview

There are hundreds of possible individual causes of confusion. Patients with acute confusion are usually elderly and often present out of hours via a call from an anxious relative or neighbour. The dementias constitute the chronic confusional states, which are not considered here.

Differential diagnosis

COMMON
- hypoxia (respiratory and cardiac)
- systemic infection
- cerebrovascular accident (CVA: stroke and transient ischaemic attack (TIA))
- hypoglycaemia
- diabetic ketoacidosis (DKA)

OCCASIONAL
- alcohol withdrawal or intoxication
- cerebral infection
- electrolyte imbalance and uraemia
- iatrogenic (e.g. digoxin, diuretics, steroids and opiates)
- myxoedema
- drug abuse

RARE
- Wernicke's encephalopathy
- cerebral tumour
- hypo- and hyperparathyroidism
- Cushing's disease
- postictal state
- carbon monoxide poisoning

Ready reckoner

	Hypoxia	Infection	CVA	Hypoglycaemia	DKA
Central cyanosis	Yes	No	No	No	No
Fever	Possible	Yes	No	No	Possible
Focal weakness	No	No	Possible	Possible	No
Ketohalitosis	No	No	No	No	Yes
Tachypnoea	Yes	Yes	No	No	Yes

Possible investigations

Acute confusion has so many causes and possible presentations that it is difficult to provide a definitive guide of investigations for the GP. A number of investigations might be considered according to the clinical picture and social circumstances; in the majority of cases, though, the patient will be admitted and necessary tests therefore arranged by the hospital.

LIKELY: urinalysis, blood sugar (usually glucometer), pulse oximetry.

POSSIBLE: FBC, CXR, ECG, cardiac enzymes, TFT.

SMALL PRINT: calcium, digoxin levels, CT scan.

- Urinalysis is very helpful if possible: look for glucose and ketones (DKA), specific gravity (dehydration), pus, blood and nitrite in UTI. Ketones alone in starvation and possibly hypoglycaemia.
- A blood glucometer reading is more practical than a formal blood glucose in the acute situation to diagnose hypo- and hyperglycaemia.
- Pulse oximetry: to detect hypoxia.
- FBC: raised WCC in infections. Raised MCV helpful pointer to excess alcohol and myxoedema.
- U&E important, especially if any signs of dehydration or on diuretics.
- LFT and TFT: alcohol, disseminated malignancy and hypothyroidism should always be considered.
- CXR: may reveal a cause of hypoxaemia (e.g. pneumonia, cardiac failure).
- ECG, cardiac enzymes: if silent infarct suspected as cause.
- Calcium: to detect possible hypo- or hyperparathyroidism.
- Digoxin levels: for digoxin toxicity.
- CT scan: invariably a hospital-based investigation in acute confusion: may reveal space-occupying lesion, bleed or infarct.

TOP TIPS

☑ The key to management is establishing that the confusion really is acute rather than a gradual deterioration of cognition. This requires a careful history from someone who knows the patient well.

☑ Don't forget a drug history: if little information is available on a visit, check the patient's medication cupboard.

☑ In acute confusional states, it can be difficult to obtain useful clinical pointers from the patient's history. The examination therefore assumes greater importance than usual.

☑ It is virtually impossible to reach a firm diagnosis and treat safely in the home. Be very sure of yourself if you choose not to admit.

☑ Central cyanosis is an ominous sign. Give oxygen, if possible, and dial 999.

☑ In a diabetic on treatment, always check the blood sugar – remember that hypoglycaemia can produce confusion with neurological signs, mimicking a CVA.

☑ Altered physiological responses in the elderly may result in a normal pulse and temperature even in the presence of significant infection. Don't be misled by this.

☑ Ask if any other household members have been unwell – carbon monoxide poisoning could affect others too.

NOTES:

DIZZINESS

The GP overview

This common and vague symptom can mean different things to different people. It is treated here as being a sense of light-headedness without the illusion of movement characteristic of vertigo. This is a useful distinction in practice as the causes of true vertigo are different – see p. 89. Dizziness tends to be a heartsink symptom as it is so common, has so many diagnostic possibilities, is so often linked with anxiety and other symptoms – and very often the exact cause remains obscure.

Differential diagnosis

COMMON
- viral illness
- anxiety (and hyperventilation)
- hypoglycaemia
- postural hypotension (e.g. elderly and pregnancy)
- vertebrobasilar insufficiency (elderly with cervical osteoarthritis)

OCCASIONAL
- acute intoxication: drugs/alcohol
- effects of chronic alcohol misuse
- iatrogenic: drug therapy (antihypertensives, antidepressants)
- cardiac arrhythmia
- any severe systemic disease

RARE
- aortic stenosis
- subclavian steal syndrome
- partial seizures
- Addison's disease
- carbon monoxide poisoning (blocked flue)

Ready reckoner

	Viral infection	Hypoglycaemia	Postural hypotension	Vertebrobasilar insufficiency	Anxiety
Sudden onset	No	Yes	Yes	Yes	No
Irritable mood	No	Possible	No	No	Possible
Episodic	No	Yes	Yes	Yes	Possible
Head turn a trigger	No	No	No	Yes	No
Relief on lying down	No	No	Yes	No	No

Possible investigations

LIKELY: none.

POSSIBLE: urinalysis, FBC, U&E, LFT, glucometer blood glucose.

SMALL PRINT: EEG, ECG/24-hour ECG, echocardiography, CT scan.

- Urinalysis for glucose: underlying diabetes may cause dizziness, either through general malaise or because of an autonomic neuropathy.
- FBC: underlying anaemia will exacerbate any cause of light-headedness; raised MCV may indicate alcohol abuse.
- U&E and LFT may be worth measuring if systemic disease suspected; in particular, sodium low, and potassium and urea both high in Addison's disease; LFT may be abnormal in alcohol abuse.
- Glucometer blood glucose: blood glucose measurement will provide a diagnosis of hypoglycaemia only if done during an episode.
- EEG: if partial epilepsy a possibility (would also then require CT scan) – both arranged by specialist.
- ECG/24 h ECG: for possible arrhythmia.
- Echocardiography: for suspected aortic stenosis.

TOP TIPS

- The first step in the history is to establish what the patient means by dizziness, and, in particular, to distinguish it from true vertigo.
- Dizziness is often multifactorial, especially in the elderly – so do not necessarily expect to find a single underlying pathology.
- If no clear diagnosis is obvious from the history, the dizziness is long standing, and the patient presents a list of other vague symptoms yet is objectively quite well (e.g. no weight loss), the likely diagnosis is anxiety.
- Don't forget that commonly prescribed drugs can cause or aggravate postural hypotension – review the patient's medication.

☑ If the patient has episodic loss of consciousness as well as dizziness, then the chances of significant pathology are much greater: investigate or refer.

☑ In puzzling cases, ask about other family members and type of domestic heating used. Carbon monoxide poisoning is a completely avoidable but regular killer.

☑ If an aortic murmur is heard, refer urgently. Significant aortic stenois can cause sudden death.

☑ Remember denial is very strong in alcoholics. If in doubt, check MCV and LFT.

NOTES:

HALLUCINATIONS

The GP overview

A hallucination is a sensory perception occurring without any external stimulus. This distinguishes it from an illusion, which is a distortion of a sensory perception. Hallucinations can occur in any sensory modality and may present in isolation or as part of a larger clinical problem (particularly an acute confusional state). A hallucination is often a very frightening experience for the sufferer.

Differential diagnosis

COMMON
- ☑ drugs (amphetamine, cocaine, LSD, ecstasy, solvents and tricyclic overdose) and drug withdrawal
- ☑ extreme fatigue
- ☑ alcoholic hallucinosis (delirium tremens of acute alcohol withdrawal)
- ☑ febrile delirium
- ☑ schizophrenia

OCCASIONAL
- ☑ severe metabolic disturbance of any cause
- ☑ temporal lobe epilepsy
- ☑ cerebral space-occupying lesion
- ☑ psychotic depression
- ☑ bereavement reaction
- ☑ hypoxia

RARE
- ☑ narcolepsy
- ☑ mania
- ☑ post-concussional state
- ☑ iatrogenic: idiosyncratic adverse drug reaction
- ☑ near-death experience

Ready reckoner

	Drugs	Fatigue	Alcohol withdrawal	Febrile delirium	Schizophrenia
Sudden onset	Yes	Possible	Yes	Yes	No
Tremor	Possible	No	Yes	Possible	No
Mainly auditory hallucination	No	No	Possible	No	Yes
Tachycardia	Possible	No	Yes	Yes	No
Cognition impaired	Yes	Possible	Yes	Yes	No

Possible investigations

The GP's use of investigations will depend on the clinical situation. If hallucinations are part of an acute confusional state, particularly in adults, admission is likely to be required and will result in a battery of tests to check, for example, for sources of fever, hypoxia and metabolic disturbance. The following are investigations the GP might use in patients who do not require admission or who are not presenting acutely.

- ☑ Urinalysis: very useful in the acute situation, particularly in the elderly. May reveal UTI or hyperglycaemic ketotic state or severe dehydration.
- ☑ Pulse oximeter: to detect hypoxia.
- ☑ Glucometer blood glucose: in a known diabetic or if any glycosuria.
- ☑ FBC and LFT: raised MCV and abnormal LFT suggest chronic alcohol excess.
- ☑ U&E: may reveal electrolyte disturbance as underlying cause.
- ☑ EEG: may suggest diagnosis of temporal lobe epilepsy or narcolepsy.
- ☑ CT scan: the definitive test for a cerebral space-occupying lesion.

TOP TIPS

- ☑ Delirium in children with a fever is quite common, especially at night and is not in itself a sinister sign; assess possible causes of the fever in the usual way, and if the cause is not serious, reassure the parents as they may be quite frightened by the child's hallucinations.
- ☑ Patients with anxiety, personality disorder and borderline mental illness may sometimes complain of auditory hallucinations, occasionally because experience has told them that this generates action from health professionals. Genuine auditory hallucinations are usually distressing and often in the second person (psychotic depression) or third person (schizophrenia) – and are accompanied by other hard evidence of mental illness.
- ☑ Minor and transient auditory and visual hallucinations are normal in the recently bereaved – but the patient will need reassurance that he or she isn't 'going mad'.

- Hallucinations caused by drugs, or by drug and alcohol withdrawal, can be terrifying and dangerous for the patient and carers, so admission is likely to be required.
- Auditory hallucinations strongly suggest psychotic illness, particularly schizophrenia and depression; visual hallucinations are almost always organic in nature.
- Purely olfactory hallucinations are pathognomic of temporal lobe pathology and require urgent investigation.
- Tactile hallucinations are very suggestive of acute alcohol withdrawal and occasionally cocaine abuse.

NOTES:

HEADACHE

The GP overview

There are almost as many causes for headache in medicine as there are disorders. This universal symptom presents a challenge to all GPs because it is common, very often non-organic, but seriously pathological just often enough to merit a thorough and usually negative examination. The chance of a sinister hidden problem is always there, but the known vast majority of benign headaches can put the clinician off guard.

Differential diagnosis

COMMON
- tension headache (underlying anxiety or depression)
- frontal sinusitis
- migraine
- cervical spondylosis
- eye strain

OCCASIONAL
- any acute febrile illness (common cause of headache but usually presents with other symptoms)
- iatrogenic (e.g. analgesic abuse, calcium antagonists, nitrates)
- chronic daily headache
- reactive hypoglycaemia
- fatigue/sleep deprivation (especially in parents)
- trigeminal, sphenopalatine and occipital neuralgias
- temporal arteritis
- post-concussional syndrome
- menstrual migraines (10–14% of women)

RARE
- cluster headache
- intracranial lesion (e.g. carcinoma, abscess, haematoma, benign intracranial hypertension)
- meningitis
- intracerebral haemorrhage
- carbon monoxide poisoning (blocked boiler flue)
- Paget's disease of skull
- severe hypertension
- pre-eclampsia

Ready reckoner

	Tension	Frontal sinusitis	Migraine	Cervical spondylosis	Eye strain
Worse on lying down	No	Yes	No	Possible	No
Congested nose	No	Yes	Possible	No	No
Worse on neck movement	No	No	Possible	Yes	No
Tender at point of pain	Possible	Yes	No	No	No
Unilateral	No	Possible	Possible	No	Possible

Possible investigations

LIKELY: none.

POSSIBLE: FBC, ESR.

SMALL PRINT: U&E, alkaline phosphatase, X-ray of sinuses, cervical spine or skull, CT scan, lumbar puncture.

- FBC: WCC raised in abscess and sinusitis. ESR essential if arteritis suspected.
- U&E: Na^+/K^+ derangement in pituitary tumours, alkaline phosphatase raised in Paget's disease.
- X-ray: may see fluid levels in sinusitis (rarely useful in diagnosis). May confirm cervical spondylosis and Paget's disease.
- CT scan: to exclude intracranial lesion.
- Lumbar puncture: in suspected meningitis; may also help in diagnosis of benign intracranial hypertension.

TOP TIPS

- Explore the patient's fears – the majority are worried about serious pathology, such as a brain tumour, and may leave the consultation dissatisfied unless this specific worry is addressed.
- Another common concern is hypertension. Patients will expect to have their blood pressure checked, even though this is almost never the cause of the symptom.
- Analgesics may paradoxically exacerbate tension headache. It is more constructive to adopt alternative approaches, such as relaxation techniques or antidepressants, as appropriate.
- Headache caused by an intracranial lesion usually produces other neurological symptoms or signs.

- Suspect subarachnoid haemorrhage given a history of sudden explosive headache. It is frequently described as 'like a blow to the head'.
- If temporal arteritis is suspected, treat immediately. The ESR provides retrospective confirmation only.
- Beware of the pregnant woman complaining of headache in the third trimester: check the blood pressure, ankles and urinalysis. Headache, particularly with visual disturbance, may be a symptom of impending eclampsia.
- A new and increasing headache present on waking and increased by stooping or straining may be due to raised intracranial pressure. Check for other symptoms and signs and refer urgently if in doubt.
- If a headache feels and smells like migraine, then it's a migraine regardless of age. However, beware of making this the diagnosis in the elderly without systematically ruling out more sinister causes first.

NOTES:

INSOMNIA

The GP overview

This problem is commoner in women, and commonest in the elderly. Normal sleep requirement varies widely. A few people need only 3–4 hours per night and the average amount of sleep needed declines with age. Self-reporting of time taken to get to sleep and hours slept are said to be inaccurate, but it is the change from the individual's normal pattern that is significant in practice.

Differential diagnosis

COMMON
- anxiety from excess psychological stress (work, relationships, finance)
- clinical depression
- chronic alcohol excess
- poor sleep hygiene: hyperstimulation (e.g. caffeine, nicotine, drugs, exciting television films) and daytime naps
- pain of chronic physical illness (e.g. osteoarthritis)

OCCASIONAL
- menopausal flushes and sweats
- nocturia
- external problems (e.g. snoring partner, children who disturb parental sleep)
- biorhythm disruption: jet lag and shift work
- respiratory problems: asthma, chronic obstructive pulmonary disease (COPD), left ventricular failure (LVF) commonest
- benzodiazepine withdrawal
- other medical problem, e.g. restless legs syndrome or GORD

RARE
- malnutrition and low body weight
- post-traumatic stress disorder
- parasomnias: nightmares, night terrors and sleepwalking
- hyperthyroidism
- mania
- sleep apnoea (usually presents as 'tired all the time' (TATT); only 30% aware of waking)

Ready reckoner

	Stress	Depression	Alcohol	Poor sleep hygiene	Pain
Slow to go off	Yes	Possible	Possible	Yes	Possible
Early morning waking	Possible	Yes	No	No	Possible
Low mood	Possible	Yes	Possible	No	Possible
Physical illness too	No	No	Possible	No	Yes
Weight loss	Possible	Possible	No	No	Possible

Possible investigations

LIKELY: none.

POSSIBLE: FBC, LFT, TFT.

SMALL PRINT: investigation of primary symptom leading to insomnia (see below).

◪ FBC (MCV), LFT and γGT may show evidence of chronic alcohol misuse.

◪ TSH will differentiate non-organic anxiety state from thyrotoxicosis.

NOTE: pain, nocturia, respiratory problems and sleep apnoea may require investigating in their own right.

TOP TIPS

◪ Uncover any underlying physical problem such as pain or nocturia and manage as appropriate – it is pointless adopting a 'sleep hygiene' approach when the problem is primarily physical.

◪ Don't forget the role of alcohol; this is often an underlying or contributory cause, paradoxically taken by the patient to relieve the insomnia.

◪ If the diagnosis seems likely to be tension or poor sleep hygiene, establish the patient's agenda early. Patients who simply want sleeping pills are unlikely to listen to well-intentioned advice until this issue has been discussed and resolved.

◪ Explain to elderly patients that sleep requirements fall with increasing age and that daytime naps are to be discouraged.

Red flags

- Shift workers are significantly at risk of developing clinical depression. Be sure to assess carefully for this pathology in the insomniac shift worker.
- Beware of young male temporary residents presenting 'urgently' with insomnia. They may well be drug addicts trying to obtain a prescription for benzodiazepines.
- Bone or joint pain waking an elderly patient at night is highly significant. In the patient with known arthritis, joint replacement may be indicated; in others, it may indicate serious bony pathology such as secondaries.
- Take the problem seriously even if the cause seems trivial or obvious (for example, a patient's snoring) – insomnia can be extremely debilitating, and by the time patients attend, they may be desperate for help.
- Anxiety and severe weight loss with sweating and tachycardia suggests hyperthyroidism. Be sure to check TSH before deciding this is non-organic.

NOTES:

LOSS OF LIBIDO

The GP overview

Loss of libido can be a daunting presentation for established GP and registrar alike. This universal problem spans adulthood in both sexes. Conventional medical school teaching seems to fail to prepare the generalist; however, the didactically taught approach of systematic enquiry and examination is the key to successful management.

Differential diagnosis

COMMON
- depression
- relationship problems
- perimenopause
- excess alcohol intake (and cirrhosis in men)
- ageing

OCCASIONAL
- low testosterone in men
- hypothyroidism
- antihypertensive treatment in men
- hyperprolactinaemic drugs in men (e.g. phenothiazines, haloperidol)
- anti-androgenic drugs in men (e.g. cimetidine, finasteride)
- anti-androgenic drugs in women (e.g. cyproterone)

RARE
- hypothalamic/pituitary disease
- renal failure
- primary testicular disease or damage
- adrenal disease (Cushing's and Addison's diseases)
- feminising tumours in men: testis or adrenal gland

Ready reckoner

	Depression	Relationship problem	Perimenopause	Alcohol	Ageing
Excessive fatigue	Yes	Possible	Yes	Possible	Possible
Irrational mood swings	Yes	Possible	Yes	Possible	No
Facial flushing	No	No	Yes	Possible	No
Alters with different partner	Possible	Yes	No	No	No
Otherwise well	No	Yes	Possible	Possible	Yes

Possible investigations

LIKELY: none.

POSSIBLE: FBC, U&E, LFT, TFT.

SMALL PRINT: hormone profile.

- ◪ FBC: may show evidence of general disease; MCV raised with significant excess alcohol.
- ◪ U&E: check for renal failure. Na$^+$ and K$^+$ deranged in adrenal disease.
- ◪ LFT and γGT: should reveal hard evidence of excess alcohol.
- ◪ TFT: will demonstrate hypothyroidism.
- ◪ Hormone profile: FSH/LH, prolactin, oestradiol and testosterone may be useful in both sexes. Altered by primary endocrine disease, drugs and alcohol.

TOP TIPS

- ◪ This is often a 'by the way' or 'while I'm here' symptom. It may be tempting to ask the patient to return for a further appointment, but bear in mind that this may mean a lost opportunity to help the patient.
- ◪ General examination is important to detect rare causes. This also demonstrates that the problem is being taken seriously.
- ◪ Avoid over-medicalising the situation if it is clearly a relationship problem.
- ◪ Be prepared to revise or augment your diagnosis – the problem is often multifactorial.
- ◪ Don't forget iatrogenic causes and be prepared to undertake a trial without treatment.

▢ Loss of libido may be the tip of the iceberg of significant pathology, such as depression or alcoholism – don't be distracted into a superficial approach.

▢ Depression and relationship difficulties can cause each other and coexist. A careful history will reveal whether antidepressants and/or psychosexual counselling is appropriate

▢ Investigations don't often help – but lower your threshold for blood tests if the patient seems generally unwell and isn't obviously depressed.

▢ Early hypothyroidism closely mimics depressive illness.

NOTES:

MEMORY LOSS

The GP overview

Memory loss is a distressing and perilous symptom for both sufferers and caring relatives. It may be due to organic or non-organic causes. Memory is classified into immediate, short-term (or recent) and long-term (or remote) memory. The type of loss varies according to the cause. Memory loss is also a feature of any cause of acute confusion; this problem is covered elsewhere (see Acute confusion, p. 68).

Differential diagnosis

COMMON
- anxiety/stress
- depressive illness
- dementia (multi-infarct, Alzheimer's disease and dementia with underlying cause, such as tumour, neurosyphilis, hypothyroidism, vitamin B_{12} and folate deficiency)
- trauma: head injury
- CVA (infarct in posterior cerebral artery territory)

OCCASIONAL
- chronic excess alcohol intake (thiamine deficiency: Korsakoff's syndrome)
- subarachnoid haemorrhage
- other thiamine deficiency: malabsorption, carcinoma stomach, hyperemesis gravidarum
- transient global amnesia
- fugue states and psychogenic amnesia
- tumour of third ventricle or hypothalamus

RARE
- personality disorder
- malingering
- intractable epilepsy
- carbon monoxide poisoning
- herpes simplex encephalitis

Ready reckoner

	Trauma	Dementia	CVA	Depression	Anxiety
Aware of problem	Possible	No	Possible	Yes	Yes
Memory loss recent events	Yes	Yes	Possible	Yes	Yes
Memory loss remote events	Possible	No	Possible	No	No
Neurological signs	Possible	Possible	Possible	No	No
Sudden onset	Yes	No	Yes	No	No

Possible investigations

LIKELY: (unless obvious depression or anxiety) FBC, TFT, LFT, calcium.

POSSIBLE: syphilis serology, B_{12} and folate levels, CT/MRI scan.

SMALL PRINT: none.

- FBC may show raised MCV, suggesting either alcohol abuse or B_{12}/folate deficiency. Check B_{12} and folate levels if MCV raised.
- TFT: hypothyroidism is an important remediable cause of dementia.
- LFT and γGT will give useful clues to alcohol intake (history likely to be unreliable).
- Calcium level: may show hypo- or hypercalcaemia.
- Syphilis serology: for possible neurosyphilis as underlying cause of dementia.
- CT scan/MRI: will detect space-occupying lesions, cerebrovascular disease, atrophy and subarachnoid haemorrhage.

TOP TIPS

- Patients with dementia are often unaware of, or deny, their memory loss; the problem is more often brought to the GP's attention by a concerned friend or relative.
- Patients who present themselves to the GP complaining of memory loss are most likely to be suffering from anxiety or depression.
- Even if a diagnosis of anxiety or depression seems obvious, patients are likely to be concerned about the possibility of dementia, which will exacerbate the situation; explaining that the problem is more to do with poor concentration than failing memory will help reassure them.
- Establishing the onset gives valuable clues to the problem: a dementia pattern progressing slowly over a year or two is likely to be Alzheimer's or multi-infarct dementia; with a shorter history, an underlying cause is possible; and sudden onset of memory loss is likely to be caused by a vascular event or trauma.
- It can be very difficult to distinguish between depression and dementia – and the two may coexist. Consider a trial of antidepressants.

☑ Rapid onset of apparent dementia over 3–6 months or less suggests a possible underlying cause.

☑ True memory loss after a head injury suggests significant trauma.

☑ Depression in the elderly may mimic dementia (pseudodementia) with behavioural changes like hoarding and bad temper. Do not miss this treatable condition.

NOTES:

VERTIGO

The GP overview

Vertigo is an illusion of movement of either the patient or his or her environment. This is both visual and positional. Associated nausea or vomiting are common and, in its acute form, it is a severe and completely disabling symptom. It must be distinguished from 'light-headedness' (see p. 71).

Differential diagnosis

COMMON
- benign positional vertigo
- vestibular migraine
- Ménière's disease
- vestibular neuritis
- Eustachian tube (ET) dysfunction (causes mild vertigo)

OCCASIONAL
- chronic otitis media
- drugs: salicylates, quinine, aminoglycosides
- acute alcohol intoxication (common, but unlikely to present to the GP)
- neurological conditions (e.g. CVA, multiple sclerosis (MS), vertebrobasilar insufficiency, syringobulbia, cerebellar tumours)
- epilepsy

RARE
- earwax (common problem but rare cause of vertigo)
- syphilis
- acoustic neuroma
- nasopharyngeal carcinoma
- post-traumatic

Ready reckoner

	Benign positional	Vestibular migraine	Ménière's	Vestibular neuritis	ET dysfunction
Tinnitus	No	No	Yes	Possible	Possible
Rapid onset, severe	Possible	Possible	Yes	Possible	No
Momentary	Yes	No	No	No	Possible
Associated viral illness	No	No	No	Yes	Possible
Recurrent	Yes	Yes	Yes	No	No

Possible investigations

There are no investigations likely to be performed in primary care. Referral might lead to a number of secondary care tests, such as audiometry for cochlear function; electronystagmography, calorimetry and brainstem-evoked responses to assess vestibular function; CT or MRI scan for possible neurological conditions; EEG for suspected epilepsy; lumbar puncture in possible MS; and syphilis serology if syphilis is suspected.

TOP TIPS

- ☑ Take a careful history: the patient may use the term 'vertigo' inaccurately, or describe true 'vertigo' as light-headedness. The diagnostic possibilities for vague dizziness and true vertigo are quite different.
- ☑ The vast majority of cases seen in primary care are benign positional vertigo, vestibular migraine, Ménière's disease or viral neuritis.
- ☑ Ménière's disease tends to be over-diagnosed. It comprises violent paroxysms of vertigo lasting for several hours, associated with deafness and tinnitus, often necessitating urgent attention because of prostration and vomiting.
- ☑ Benign positional vertigo is usually easily diagnosed by the history: the patient experiences vertigo lasting only for a few seconds, classically on turning over in bed.
- ☑ Vestibular migraine is under-diagnosed. Consider it in any case of recurrent vertigo – enquire about headache before, during or after the vertigo.

☑ The patient who has chronic otitis media and then develops vertigo probably has significant disease – especially if the fistula sign is positive (putting pressure on the external ear canal by forcibly occluding the external auditory meatus with a finger causes vertigo). Refer urgently.

☑ Young or middle-aged patients with atypical, episodic vertigo who have other, diffuse and transient neurological symptoms may have MS.

☑ Loss of consciousness with vertigo suggests epilepsy.

☑ An acoustic neuroma can cause quite mild vertigo. Consider this possibility if the patient also has a unilateral sensorineural deafness and tinnitus.

☑ A neurological cause such as a stroke is suggested by any CNS symptoms or signs; a new type of headache, especially occipital; acute deafness (otherwise unexplained); or vertical nystagmus.

NOTES:

CHEST

Acute shortness of breath

Chest pain

Chronic shortness of breath

Cough in adults

Cough in children

Coughing up blood

Palpitations

ACUTE SHORTNESS OF BREATH

The GP overview

This is a terrifying symptom for the patient, and the subjective feeling of shortness of breath is not predictably related to the type or degree of pathology. This, combined with the fact that the cause is often organic, means that a careful and urgent assessment is mandatory.

Differential diagnosis

COMMON
- asthma
- pneumonia
- acute LVF
- acute exacerbation of COPD
- hyperventilation

OCCASIONAL
- pneumothorax
- pulmonary embolism
- pleural effusion
- diabetic ketoacidosis (DKA)
- lobar collapse (tumour)

RARE
- aspiration pneumonitis
- Guillain–Barré syndrome
- hypovolaemic shock
- shock lung (adult respiratory distress syndrome)
- laryngeal obstruction

Ready reckoner

	Asthma	Pneumonia	LVF	Exacerbation of COPD	Hyperventilation
Purulent phlegm	Possible	Yes	No	Yes	No
Coarse crackles	No	Yes	No	Yes	No
Bilateral wheeze	Yes	No	Possible	Yes	No
Bilateral fine crackles	No	No	Yes	Possible	No
Focal reduced air entry	No	Yes	No	No	No

Possible investigations

The GP is highly unlikely to initiate any investigations at all. If the patient with acute shortness of breath is ill enough – or the diagnosis obscure enough – to warrant investigation, then the patient probably requires admission. The following therefore refers to those few cases in which the patient is reasonably well, the diagnosis unclear and the scenario not so urgent that immediate referral is required.

- Urinalysis: glucose and ketones in DKA. Confirm with a glucometer reading.
- Sputum culture: very occasionally helpful in infective processes not settling with first-line empirical treatment.
- FBC: WCC raised in infection. Anaemia may be significant incidental finding.
- Pulse oximetry – hypoxia suggests a significant problem.
- CXR an essential part of assessment but usually done after admission/referral.
- Other investigations such as blood gases and ventilation/perfusion scans might be required to clinch a diagnosis but would be arranged by the admitting team.

TOP TIPS

- If the diagnosis is likely to be hyperventilation, instruct the patient to rebreathe from a paper bag while waiting for you. This action may curtail the attack by the time you arrive.
- Spacer devices can be as effective as nebulisers when managing acute exacerbations of asthma, and are more practical to use when on call.
- Sudden onset of breathlessness in an elderly patient in the middle of the night is likely to be LVF. Remember that it may be have been precipitated by an infarct.

Red flags

- ☑ Cyanosis is an ominous sign meriting a 'blue light' ambulance and oxygen as soon as possible.
- ☑ The presence of intercostal recession and use of accessory muscles of respiration indicate severe respiratory distress whatever the aetiology. Admit.
- ☑ If a foreign body has been inhaled, astute telephone assessment and clear, calm advice may be lifesaving.
- ☑ Acute confusion with breathlessness indicates severe hypoxaemia, metabolic disturbance or sepsis. Admit urgently.
- ☑ Don't forget that pneumothorax is commoner in asthmatics – consider this diagnosis if an asthmatic suddenly becomes more short of breath.

NOTES:

CHEST PAIN

The GP overview

Acute chest pain is a regular visitor to general practice: it may generate more adrenaline in the physician than the patient. In spite of a constellation of causes, a good basic clinical approach will determine the diagnosis in nearly all cases, long before any necessary investigations are complete.

Differential diagnosis

COMMON

- angina/MI
- GORD
- anxiety (Da Costa's syndrome)
- pulled muscle
- Tietze's syndrome (costochondritis)

OCCASIONAL

- pleurisy
- peptic ulcer
- biliary colic
- shingles
- mastitis
- Bornholm disease

RARE

- pulmonary infarct
- hypertrophic obstructive cardiomyopathy
- pericarditis
- fractured ribs
- myocarditis
- pneumothorax
- dissecting aortic aneurysm

Ready reckoner

	Angina	GORD	Anxiety	Pulled muscle	Tietze's syndrome
Worse on exertion	Yes	Possible	Possible	Possible	Possible
Worse lying down	No	Yes	Possible	No	No
Eased by rest	Yes	Possible	Possible	Yes	Possible
Chest tenderness	No	No	Possible	Yes	Yes
Swelling at tender point	No	No	No	No	Yes

Possible investigations

LIKELY: ECG.

POSSIBLE: FBC, CXR, pulse oximetry, secondary care cardiac investigations, OGD, ultrasound of abdomen.

SMALL PRINT: Helicobacter tests, ventilation/perfusion scan (hospital-based).

- ECG: may show evidence of cardiac ischaemia, pericarditis or pulmonary embolism.
- FBC: WCC raised in pleurisy and may be raised in Tietze's syndrome.
- CXR: may reveal chest infection, rib fracture, heart disease, cardiomyopathy or pneumothorax.
- Pulse oximetry: hypoxia a sign of significant cardiac or respiratory problem in the acute setting.
- Secondary care cardiac investigations: to clarify whether a cardiac cause.
- Ultrasound of abdomen: to check for gallstones.
- OGD: to confirm peptic ulcer or oesophagitis.
- *Helicobacter* tests useful in the presence of duodenal ulcer.
- Ventilation/perfusion scan (in hospital): to confirm pulmonary infarction.

TOP TIPS

- The history is all-important and will usually provide the diagnosis. Except in an obvious emergency, take your time getting the facts straight.
- If you feel worried enough to obtain an urgent ECG then you ought to consider whether the patient really requires an urgent medical opinion or admission.
- Watching the patient's hand as the symptoms are being described can provide very helpful clues. A clenched fist on the chest is worrying; a single pointing finger much less so.
- Musculoskeletal pain and pleurisy both cause pain on deep inspiration – but the former usually also displays muscle or rib tenderness.
- Tietze's syndrome is distinguished from costochondritis by the presence of a palpable swelling, caused by oedema, at the site of maximal tenderness. However, management is largely the same.
- Always encourage the patient to contact you if the problem persists or deteriorates.
- If in doubt, play safe: give aspirin (if not allergic) and admit.

- Don't delay if the symptoms clearly suggest an infarct; admit the patient (via the telephone if necessary).
- A normal ECG does not exclude an infarct. Treat the patient, not the test.
- Symptoms of genuine and significant pathology may be clouded by various ensuing anxiety symptoms. Take time to tease them out.
- Performing unnecessary tests when the diagnosis is clearly anxiety is likely to exacerbate the situation.
- If the diagnosis remains unclear, examine the abdomen, especially for significant epigastric tenderness.

NOTES:

CHRONIC SHORTNESS OF BREATH

The GP overview

Shortness of breath is defined as difficult, laboured breathing. Medical teaching tends to focus on individual pathologies; however, in practice there is often some overlap between several contributory causes and sometimes the diagnosis can only be made after therapeutic trials of treatment.

Differential diagnosis

COMMON
- obesity/unfitness
- COPD
- anaemia
- congestive cardiac failure (CCF)
- asthma

OCCASIONAL
- bronchiectasis
- recurrent pulmonary emboli
- bronchial carcinoma with lobar collapse
- pleural effusion
- aortic stenosis
- chronic hyperventilation

RARE
- pulmonary fibrosis
- large hiatus hernia
- fibrosing alveolitis
- undiagnosed congenital heart disease
- neurological: motor neurone disease and the muscular dystrophies
- sarcoidosis
- extrinsic allergic alveolitis (bird fancier's lung etc.)

Ready reckoner

	Obesity/unfitness	COPD	Anaemia	CCF	Asthma
Worse lying down	Possible	No	No	Yes	No
Swelling of ankles	No	Possible	No	Yes	No
Cough	No	Yes	No	Yes	Yes
Copious sputum	No	Yes	No	Yes	Possible
Pallor	No	No	Yes	No	No

Possible investigations

LIKELY: CXR, FBC.

POSSIBLE: peak flow, U&E, LFT, ESR/CRP, BNP, ECG, spirometry.

SMALL PRINT: pulse oximetry, CT scan, V/Q scan, pleural tap, echocardiogram, Kveim test.

- CXR: the single most useful investigation. Will reveal or give clues to many of the causes listed.
- FBC essential to look for anaemia; ESR/CRP raised in carcinoma, inflammation and infection.
- U&E and LFT: impaired renal function will contribute to CCF; LFT may show signs of disseminated carcinoma.
- Peak expiratory flow rate variability in asthma; more comprehensive lung function tests (spirometry) are more helpful to diagnose COPD and other lung diseases.
- ECG: heart failure is unlikely if the ECG is normal.
- BNP: likely to be elevated in heart failure.
- Pulse oximetry: helps guide assessment of severity and decisions about oxygen therapy but of little help in making the diagnosis.
- Referral for more difficult cases may result in CT or V/Q scans (e.g. for bronchiectasis or pulmonary emboli), pleural tap (diagnostic and therapeutic for pleural effusion), echocardiography (for heart valve lesions and assessment of left ventricular function) and Kveim test (for sarcoidosis).

TOP TIPS

- Cardiac failure may arise as a complication of COPD. Remember this possibility if a patient with COPD complains of gradually increasing breathlessness unrelieved by standard treatment.
- Cases of breathlessness in the elderly may be multifactorial and difficult to diagnose precisely even after investigation. Do not underestimate the value of a trial of treatment, e.g. a course of steroids for possible asthma or potential reversibility in COPD.
- In the young and middle-aged, sighing speech and shortness of breath worse with stress or

without any clear pattern – especially if the patient does not consistently have a problem with exercise – are likely to be caused by hyperventilation.

Red flags

- ◪ Weight loss and clubbing with shortness of breath suggest bronchial carcinoma, though bronchiectasis is possible – arrange an urgent CXR.
- ◪ Wheeze may be present in cardiac failure – crepitations may not. Look for other signs of CCF in the elderly and consider appropriate investigation and treatment.
- ◪ Remember that acute causes can supervene at any time: for example, beware of pneumothorax in the asthmatic
- ◪ Cardiac failure has a poor prognosis; look for an underlying cause (e.g. hypertension) and consider echocardiography with a view to starting ACE inhibitors.
- ◪ Don't forget anaemia as a possible cause – contrary to popular belief this tends to cause shortness of breath rather than tiredness.

NOTES:

COUGH IN ADULTS

The GP overview

This is a symptom that patients seem to fear or value – as a signifier of possible cancer or a justifier of antibiotics – far more than GPs. Most coughs are simply viral URTIs, but the GP should be aware of the various other possibilities, especially when the symptom is persistent.

Differential diagnosis

COMMON
- URTI
- LRTI
- asthma
- COPD
- ACE inhibitor side effect

OCCASIONAL
- smoking (including passive smoking)
- lung tumour (primary or secondary)
- rhinitis
- GORD
- LVF
- bronchiectasis
- aspiration (e.g. post stroke)

RARE
- TB
- other medication side effect (e.g. methotrexate)
- pulmonary fibrosis
- fibrosing alveolitis
- extrinsic allergic alveolitis
- psychogenic
- laryngeal carcinoma
- inhaled foreign body
- diaphragmatic irritation (e.g. abscess)

Ready reckoner

	URTI	LRTI	Asthma	COPD	ACE inhibitor side effect
Associated shortness of breath	No	Possible	Possible	Yes	No
Productive cough	Possible	Yes	Possible	Yes	No
Persistent or recurrent cough	No	No	Yes	Yes	Yes
Audible wheeze	No	Possible	Possible	Possible	No
On ACE inhibitor	Possible	Possible	Possible	Possible	Yes

Possible investigations

LIKELY: none.

POSSIBLE: FBC, ESR/CRP, spirometry, PEFR.

SMALL PRINT: sputum, cardiac investigations, serum precipitins, hospital-based investigations such as CT scan and bronchoscopy.

- FBC: Hb may be reduced in malignancy and chronic illness; WCC raised in infections, eosinophils raised in allergic conditions.
- ESR/CRP: raised in neoplasia, infective and inflammatory conditions.
- CXR: may show signs in a variety of the relevant differentials, such as LRTI, tumour and TB.
- Spirometry: may show characteristic patterns particularly in asthma, COPD and pulmonary fibrosis.
- Serial peak flow: may be helpful in diagnosis of asthma.
- Sputum: may be useful in diagnosing TB and occasionally helps guide antibiotic treatment in LRTI or exacerbation of COPD.
- Cardiac investigations: such as BNP or echocardiogram if LVF suspected.
- Serum precipitins: in suspected extrinsic allergic alveolitis.
- Hospital-based investigations: further investigations such as CT scan or bronchoscopy be required to clarify CXR abnormalities or pursue clinical suspicion.

TOP TIPS

- Explain to patients that it is not unusual for the cough of a simple URTI to go on for 3 weeks – this will reduce unnecessary re-attendances.
- Take a careful history of provoking factors in the case of persistent cough – this is more likely to reveal the diagnosis than is chest auscultation.
- Have a low threshold for arranging a CXR in the middle-aged and elderly smoker with a cough.

- ACE inhibitor-associated cough may come on many months – or even longer – after initiating treatment. It starts to improve within 1–4 weeks of stopping treatment but may take 3 months to settle completely.
- In a persistent cough with a normal CXR and no chest signs, think asthma, GORD and rhinitis – a therapeutic trial for each may be needed to clinch the diagnosis.

- Remember to ask about foreign travel. Atypical pneumonias are infrequent, and TB rare, but both can still present.
- Beware of persistent cough, weight loss and voice change in a smoker – arrange an X-ray to exclude malignancy.
- Night sweats with persistent cough suggest significant pathology such as TB or malignancy.
- Beware the patient on immunosuppressants: these drugs may alter the clinical picture, predispose to serious complications and in some cases (e.g. methotrexate) may be the cause of the cough itself.

NOTES:

COUGH IN CHILDREN

The GP overview

The symptom GPs love to hate because it can appear so trivial. Reassurance and explanation are often all that is required, and this can build a bond with parents and children. Take parents seriously and sympathetically: nocturnal cough is a destroyer of sleep and family peace.

Differential diagnosis

COMMON
- URTI
- LRTI
- post-nasal drip (e.g. post URTI, allergic rhinitis)
- asthma
- pertussis

OCCASIONAL
- inhaled foreign body
- GORD
- psychogenic

RARE
- TB
- cystic fibrosis
- earwax or foreign body in the ear canal
- immune deficiency
- interstitial lung disease
- congenital, e.g. trachea-oesophageal fistula

Ready reckoner

	URTI	LRTI	PN drip	Asthma	Pertussis
Child unwell	No	Possible	No	Possible	Possible
Chest signs	No	Yes	No	Possible	No
Spring/summer exacerbation	No	No	Possible	Possible	No
Marked nasal catarrh	Yes	No	Yes	Possible	No
Cough >3 weeks	No	Possible	Possible	Yes	Yes

Possible investigations

LIKELY: none.

POSSIBLE: FBC, ESR/CRP, CXR, serial peak flow or spirometry.

SMALL PRINT: pertussis serology, sweat test, secondary care investigations (e.g. for interstitial lung disease or immune deficiency).

- ▱ FBC, ESR/CRP: WCC raised in infection – marked lymphocytosis in pertussis; ESR/CRP elevated in any inflammatory process.
- ▱ CXR: may be helpful in LRTI, TB, inhaled foreign body, cystic fibrosis.
- ▱ Serial peak flow or spirometry: to help confirm a diagnosis of asthma.
- ▱ Pertussis serology: if a clinical suspicion of pertussis needs confirming.
- ▱ Sweat test: for cystic fibrosis.
- ▱ Other secondary care investigations: may be required after referral (e.g. for interstitial lung disease or immune deficiency).

TOP TIPS

- ▱ Think pertussis in any paroxysmal cough lasting more than 3 weeks – it is much more common than most people, and many doctors, realise.
- ▱ Educate parents about the likely duration of URTI-related coughs and simple measures to take. Avoid prescribing, as this simply reinforces the tendency to attend the doctor for minor, self-limiting illness.
- ▱ In the asthmatic child, a cough may be a sign of poor control: check treatment, compliance and inhaler technique.
- ▱ Many parents panic that a cough might harm their child. An explanation that a cough is often simply a way of 'keeping the lungs clear' can defuse the situation.
- ▱ An aural foreign body is an unusual but remediable cause of childhood cough.

Red flags

- ☑ Parents tend to focus on the cough. In the acute situation, rather more important are symptoms and signs of respiratory distress – the NICE traffic light system for febrile children is useful in the acutely coughing febrile child and will help guide the need for admission.
- ☑ A dramatic and abrupt onset of coughing in a child should make you consider an inhaled foreign body.
- ☑ Beware the 'poorly controlled asthmatic' who isn't thriving – this could be cystic fibrosis.

NOTES:

COUGHING UP BLOOD

The GP overview

Patients invariably view this relatively uncommon symptom as representing something serious – this is rarely the case in primary care. In practice, the origin of the blood may not be immediately obvious: quite often, blood from the nose or throat may be coughed out with saliva (spurious haemoptysis) and described as 'coughing up blood'.

Differential diagnosis

COMMON

- chest infection
- pulmonary embolism (PE)
- bronchogenic carcinoma
- pulmonary oedema
- prolonged coughing

OCCASIONAL

- bronchiectasis
- mitral stenosis
- polyarteritis nodosa
- tuberculosis
- tumour of larynx or trachea

RARE

- associated with SLE
- aspergillosis
- Goodpasture's syndrome
- contusion due to trauma
- pulmonary arteriovenous malformations (50% associated with hereditary haemorrhagic telangiectasia)

Ready reckoner

	Chest infection	PE	Bronchogenic carcinoma	Pulmonary oedema	Prolonged coughing
Purulent sputum	Yes	No	Possible	No	Possible
Pink frothy sputum	No	No	No	Yes	No
Chest signs	Yes	Possible	Possible	Possible	No
SOB	Yes	Yes	Possible	Yes	No
Fever	Yes	Possible	Possible	No	No

Possible investigations

LIKELY: CXR.

POSSIBLE: FBC, ESR/CRP, autoantibody screen, sputum, pulse oximetry.

SMALL PRINT: bronchoscopy, ventilation/perfusion scan, echocardiogram, other chest imaging (e.g. CT scan).

- CXR: this is the single most valuable investigation for detecting many of the causes listed.
- Sputum microbiology: may be needed to look for acid-fast bacilli of TB.
- FBC and ESR/CRP: for anaemia (LVF and malignant disease); WCC raised in infection, ESR/CRP raised in malignancy, infection and inflammatory conditions.
- Autoantibody screen: for assessing possible connective tissue disease.
- Pulse oximetry: hypoxia points to significant acute lung pathology.
- Hospital-based tests: various other investigations may be considered according to the likely aetiology and would usually be arranged by the hospital specialist after referral, e.g. bronchoscopy, ventilation/perfusion scan, CT scan and echocardiography.

TOP TIPS

- In younger patients, the symptom is most commonly caused by vigorous coughing. If this is clearly the case, and the haemoptysis was minor, do not engender unnecessary anxiety by arranging a CXR.
- Take a careful history. The terminology used by some patients can confuse the doctor as to whether blood was coughed or vomited up.
- Don't forget that most patients – and smokers in particular – will be worried that the symptom represents cancer. Reassure firmly when appropriate, but investigate early those cases that concern you, providing an adequate explanation as to why you are arranging a CXR and making firm arrangements for follow-up.

- Any smoker with significant haemoptysis should have a CXR – particularly if there are other sinister features such as shortness of breath, weight loss, persistent cough or clubbing.
- PE causes sudden onset of shortness of breath with pleuritic pain. Consider this diagnosis if there is no other obvious explanation for the symptoms, especially if the patient has a tachycardia. Signs of DVT may only appear later, or sometimes never at all.
- TB is on the increase in the UK. Consider this possibility in the elderly, immigrants and vagrants. It often mimics malignancy.
- If haemoptysis persists, arrange referral even if the CXR is clear – some lesions may not appear on the X-ray, or may only develop after some time has elapsed. Other investigations may be required.

NOTES:

PALPITATIONS

The GP overview

Palpitations are presented fairly frequently to the GP, sometimes in isolation but more often immersed in other symptoms. Patients use the word 'palpitations' to describe a remarkable variety of sensations, and it is important to establish exactly what is meant. Cardiac causes are rare; anxiety about a cardiac problem, and anxiety as a cause of the symptom, are common.

Differential diagnosis

COMMON
- anxiety (increased awareness of normal heartbeat)
- sinus tachycardia (e.g. stress, fever, exercise)
- atrial ectopics
- ventricular ectopics
- supraventricular tachycardia (SVT)

OCCASIONAL
- thyrotoxicosis (combination of sinus tachycardia and increased awareness even if ventricular ectopics are absent)
- menopause (due to sudden vasodilation)
- atrial fibrillation (AF – various causes, e.g. IHD, mitral valve disease, alcohol)
- iatrogenic (e.g. digoxin, nifedipine)
- atrial flutter

RARE
- heart block (especially with changes in block)
- sick sinus syndrome
- drug abuse
- ventricular tachycardia (VT)

Ready reckoner

	Anxiety	Sinus tachycardia	Atrial ectopics	Ventricular ectopics	SVT
Sudden onset	Possible	No	Possible	Possible	Yes
'Heart racing'	Yes	Yes	No	No	Yes
'Heart misses a beat'	Possible	No	Yes	Yes	No
Underlying heart disease	No	No	No	Possible	Possible
Rate/rhythm abnormal during episode	No	Yes	Yes	Yes	Yes

Possible investigations

LIKELY: ECG, TFT.

POSSIBLE: U&E, 24 h ECG or event monitor.

SMALL PRINT: further investigation to establish underlying cause.

- ◪ ECG: may show arrhythmia itself or evidence of ischaemic heart disease or Wolff–Parkinson–White syndrome.
- ◪ TFT: thyrotoxicosis can cause palpitations or exacerbate other causes.
- ◪ U&E: electrolyte disturbance can precipitate or aggravate some arrhythmias.
- ◪ 24 h ECG or event monitor: to provide ECG evidence of the arrhythmia.
- ◪ Further investigation of underlying cause: e.g. stress test for ischaemic heart disease, echocardiography for valve disease.

TOP TIPS

- ◪ Take time to obtain a clear history, as the patient's perception of a 'palpitation' may differ markedly from yours.
- ◪ In paroxysmal cases, suggest that the patient attends the surgery or casualty urgently during an attack to obtain an ECG.
- ◪ Patients can easily be taught to take their own pulse. Self-reported pulse rates can help considerably in establishing a diagnosis.
- ◪ Most patients with palpitations fear heart disease, and this anxiety exacerbates the symptoms. Ensure this fear is resolved whenever possible.

- Multiple, or multifocal, ventricular ectopics suggest significant ischaemic heart disease – and may herald VT or fibrillation if they follow an infarct.
- Sudden onset of tachycardia in a young adult with breathlessness, dizziness, chest pain and polyuria suggests significant SVT.
- Patients complaining of palpitations who are in AF are likely to have paroxysmal or recent onset AF, with significant risk of systemic embolism. Consider urgent referral for anticoagulation.
- Remember that digoxin can aggravate as well as resolve some arrhythmias.

NOTES:

EAR

Deafness

Earache

Ear discharge

Tinnitus

DEAFNESS

The GP overview

Deafness is a frustrating symptom. In children it creates educational difficulties and parental worry. In adults, everyday life is fraught with difficulties, and there may be stigmatisation. Three million adults in the UK suffer some degree of persistent deafness. Congenital causes acquired in utero are not included here.

Differential diagnosis

COMMON
- earwax
- otitis media (OM)
- otitis externa (OE)
- glue ear (serous otitis media)/Eustachian dysfunction
- presbyacusis (senile deafness)

OCCASIONAL
- Ménière's disease
- otosclerosis
- noise damage to cochlea
- barotrauma
- viral acoustic neuritis
- large nasal polyps or nasopharyngeal tumour
- drugs: streptomycin, gentamicin, aspirin overdose

RARE
- vascular (haemorrhage, thrombosis of cochlear vessels)
- acoustic neuroma
- vitamin B_{12} deficiency
- CNS causes (e.g. multiple sclerosis, cerebral secondary carcinoma)
- cholesteatoma
- Paget's disease
- traumatic (e.g. to tympanic membrane or ossicles)

Ready reckoner

	Earwax	OM	OE	Glue ear/ET	Presbyacusis
Pain	Possible	Yes	Yes	No	No
Pinna traction painful	No	No	Yes	No	No
Discharge from EAM	Possible	Possible	Yes	No	No
Conductive deafness	Yes	Yes	Yes	Yes	No
Fluid level on drum	No	No	No	Yes	No

Possible investigations

LIKELY: (in children) audiogram and tympanometry.

POSSIBLE: ear swab.

SMALL PRINT: FBC/B_{12} levels, skull X-ray, further imaging.

- ▰ Audiometry quantifies loss and distinguishes sensorineural from conductive hearing loss.
- ▰ Tympanometry measures the compliance of the eardrum. Fluid in the middle ear flattens the compliance curve.
- ▰ Swab of ear discharge: discharge can be swabbed to guide treatment in refractory otitis externa.
- ▰ FBC/B_{12} levels: to confirm B_{12} deficiency.
- ▰ Skull X-ray: for Paget's disease.
- ▰ Further imaging: e.g. CT and MRI scans may be arranged by specialist for suspected acoustic neuroma, multiple sclerosis or cerebral pathology.

TOP TIPS

- ▰ Take parents seriously if they suspect their child is deaf. There may be no physical signs in glue ear, and tympanometry will yield the diagnosis.
- ▰ Warn patients with otitis media that hearing may take a few weeks to return completely to normal – this saves unnecessary attendances with patients complaining that 'The antibiotics haven't worked'.
- ▰ In a case with no immediately alarming features and no past history of significant ear disease, it is reasonable to defer a comprehensive history and examination – instead, take a quick look at the ear canals. If the diagnosis appears to be earwax, arrange syringing. Assess in more detail only if there is no earwax or syringing doesn't solve the problem.
- ▰ Remember how to perform and interpret Rinne's and Weber's tests – these are invaluable in assessing the less straightforward cases.

- Remember the possibility of acoustic neuroma if there is progressive unilateral sensorineural deafness – especially if there is accompanying tinnitus, vertigo or neurological symptoms or signs.
- Otherwise unexplained and persistent serous otitis media in adults may be due to nasopharyngeal carcinoma – refer for urgent examination of the nasopharyngeal space.
- Sudden onset of profound sensorineural deafness is usually viral or vascular and requires same-day ENT assessment.
- Otosclerosis requires early diagnosis for effective treatment. Consider the diagnosis in otherwise unexplained conductive deafness in young adults, especially if there is a family history.

NOTES:

EARACHE

The GP overview

This the commonest reason for an out-of-hours call for a child. Parental distress is often as great as the child's, and appropriate advice can do much to relieve this – even over the telephone. Causes in adults are far more varied than for children and can originate in the pinna, ear canal, middle ear and from neighbouring structures (referred pain).

Differential diagnosis

COMMON
- infective otitis media (OM): bacterial/viral
- infective otitis externa (OE): bacterial/fungal/viral
- boils and furuncles of the canal and pinna
- trauma (especially cotton buds) and foreign bodies (including earwax)
- throat problems: tonsillitis/pharyngitis/quinsy

OCCASIONAL
- temporomandibular joint (TMJ) dysfunction
- dental abscess
- impacted molar
- trigeminal neuralgia
- ear canal eczema/seborrhoeic dermatitis
- chondrodermatitis nodularis helicis externa

RARE
- mastoiditis
- cervical spondylosis
- cholesteatoma
- malignant disease
- barotrauma

Ready reckoner

	OM	OE	Boils	Trauma	Throat problems
Discharge	Possible	Yes	Possible	Possible	No
Pain on pulling pinna and pressing tragus	No	Yes	Yes	Possible	No
Red, bulging eardrum	Yes	No	No	No	No
Deafness	Yes	Possible	No	Possible	No
Pain on swallowing	No	No	No	No	Yes

Possible investigations

LIKELY: none.

POSSIBLE: ear swab.

SMALL PRINT: X-rays of TMJ, teeth and mastoid bone, FBC, Paul–Bunnell test.

- Swab of ear canal useful if discharge present, after failure of empirical first-line treatment.
- X-ray of mastoid bone excludes mastoiditis if mastoid clear – usually arranged by specialist. X-rays of TMJ and teeth are the remit of the dentist or oral surgeon.
- FBC and Paul–Bunnell test useful if glandular fever suspected. The diagnosis provides a label and guides further advice, though no specific treatment exists.
- Further specialist investigations may include CT/MRI as the only way adequately (non-invasively) to investigate the inner ear and temporal bone anatomy.

TOP TIPS

- Persistent debris in the ear canal will prevent resolution of OE and mask possible underlying causes. Aural toilet is essential.
- If inserting the aural speculum causes pain, the diagnosis is likely to be otitis externa or a furuncle.
- Don't forget to ask about trauma – especially the use of a cotton bud. Excavating earwax with a bud tends to produce an inflamed canal and drum, mimicking infection.
- Earache can be excruciating – don't underestimate the need for adequate analgesia while you establish and treat the cause.

☑ Consider mastoiditis if foul-smelling discharge is present for more than 10 days. Look for swelling behind the ear and downward displacement of the pinna.

☑ Don't be too ready to diagnose otitis media in children – URTIs and crying inevitably result in some redness of the drum. Indiscriminate prescribing may lead to iatrogenic problems or the masking of the true diagnosis.

☑ Beware the elderly patient with intractable, unexplained earache – refer to exclude a nasopharyngeal carcinoma.

NOTES:

EAR DISCHARGE

The GP overview

This is often seen in swimmers and returned tropical travellers. It is frequently a sequel to water trapped behind earwax in the ear canal, which swells and encourages stasis and subsequent infection. The vast majority of cases seen settle with simple treatment, but be wary of rarer serious causes.

Differential diagnosis

COMMON
- boil
- acute suppurative otitis media (OM)
- infective otitis externa (OE): viral, bacterial and fungal
- chronic suppurative otitis media
- reactive otitis externa: seborrhoeic dermatitis, eczema, psoriasis

OCCASIONAL
- cholesteatoma
- trauma: often a result of over-vigorous attempts to clean the ear
- bullous myringitis (otitis externa haemorrhagica)
- infection with foreign body (insects, beads in toddlers)
- liquefying excess earwax

RARE
- mastoiditis
- necrotising (or malignant) otitis externa
- squamous and basal cell (rarer) carcinoma of the EAM
- keratosis obturans (bolus of abnormally desquamated epithelium and earwax: associated with chronic bronchitis and bronchiectasis)
- herpes zoster oticus
- cerebrospinal fluid (CSF) otorrhoea

Ready reckoner

	Boil	OM	Infective OE	Chronic OM	Reactive OE
Painless	No	No	Possible	Yes	Possible
Other skin disease	Possible	No	No	No	Yes
Tender tragus	Yes	No	Yes	No	Yes
Drum perforated	No	Yes	No	Yes	No
Ipsilateral deafness	No	Yes	Possible	Yes	Possible

Possible investigations

LIKELY: none.

POSSIBLE: swab, urinalysis.

SMALL PRINT: skull/mastoid X-rays, CT or MRI scan, audiometry.

- Swab of ear discharge: helps guide treatment in refractory cases.
- Urine for glucose: to exclude underlying diabetes if infections are recurrent (especially boils).
- X-ray of the mastoid process will show a cloudy appearance in the mastoid air cells in mastoiditis.
- CT or MRI scan is the best way to investigate possible invasion of temporal bone by tumour, cholesteatoma.
- Audiometry may be required to assess baseline hearing loss in chronic OM, so improvement after definitive surgical treatment can be measured.
- Skull X-ray: may show middle cranial fossa fracture in CSF otorrhoea (performed in hospital after significant trauma).

TOP TIPS

- Otitis externa is often recurrent: to minimise future problems, advise the patient to avoid getting water in the ear and stop using cotton buds. Also treat any underlying skin disease.
- In the presence of ear discharge, pain on moving the tragus suggests otitis externa or a boil; in the case of the former, the patient tends to present with itching rather than pain.
- Most cases of otitis externa and media settle with empirical treatment and so don't require a swab. Only investigate if they do not respond to first-line treatment.
- If the diagnosis is not certain, be sure to follow up after initial treatment to visualise the drum; if persistent discharge makes this impossible, refer to the ENT outpatients department for aural toilet and further assessment.

Red flags

☑ Heat, tenderness and swelling over the mastoid process suggests mastoiditis: refer urgently.

☑ If ear discharge does not clear with usual therapy, refer for microsuction of debris (aural toilet) to speed resolution and exclude significant middle-ear disease.

☑ Very rarely, middle-ear infection causing discharge can progress centrally, causing, for example, meningitis or cerebral abscess – so refer immediately any patient with ear discharge who becomes confused or develops neurological signs.

☑ The use of aminoglycoside or polymyxin drops in the presence of a perforated tympanic membrane carries a risk of ototoxicity (though some specialists do use such drops even if perforation is present). When using potentially ototoxic drops, be as certain as you can about what you are treating.

☑ Beware severe otitis externa in elderly diabetics – it may be the necrotising ('malignant') form.

NOTES:

TINNITUS

The GP overview

This means noises heard (nearly always subjectively) in the ears or head. They are often described as being like a whistling kettle, an engine, or in time with the heartbeat. As a short-lived phenomenon, it is very common (often with URTIs) – such cases do not usually present to the GP. More serious, persistent tinnitus occurs in up to 2% of the population. It is very distressing and can cause secondary depression and insomnia. Objective tinnitus is very rare.

Differential diagnosis

COMMON
- earwax
- hearing loss (20% of cases: chronic noise damage and presbyacusis)
- suppurative otitis media (also chronic infection and serous OM)
- otosclerosis
- Ménière's disease

OCCASIONAL
- after a sudden loud noise (e.g. gunfire)
- head injury (especially basal skull fracture)
- impacted wisdom teeth and TMJ dysfunction
- drugs: aspirin overdose, loop diuretics, aminoglycosides, quinine
- hypertension and atherosclerosis

RARE
- acoustic neuroma
- palatal myoclonus (objectively detectable)
- arteriovenous fistulae and arterial bruits (objectively detectable)
- severe anaemia and renal failure
- glomus jugulare tumours (objectively detectable)

Ready reckoner

	Earwax	Hearing loss	Otitis media	Otosclerosis	Ménière's disease
Sudden onset	Yes	No	Yes	No	Possible
Pain in ear	Possible	No	Yes	No	No
Rinne's test positive	No	Yes	Possible	No	Yes
Vertigo	Possible	No	Possible	No	Yes
High-pitched	No	Possible	No	No	Yes

Possible investigations

LIKELY: none.

POSSIBLE: tympanogram, audiogram, MRI scan (all usually in secondary care).

SMALL PRINT: FBC, U&E, skull X-ray, angiography (the latter two in secondary care).

- FBC and U&E: if anaemia or renal failure suspected.
- Tympanogram for middle-ear function and stapedial reflex threshold. Audiogram to assess hearing loss objectively.
- Cerebral angiography: if vascular pathology suspected.
- MRI scan: the most sensitive way to examine the inner ear and skull for structural lesions.
- Skull X-ray: if associated with significant head injury.

TOP TIPS

- Most patients are afraid of the diagnosis of tinnitus because of its potentially debilitating nature. If the cause is clearly self-limiting or remediable, take time to reassure the patient.
- Have a low threshold for referral in persistent tinnitus. While no specific treatment may be available, this shows that you are taking the problem seriously, ensures that remediable problems won't be missed and may give the patient access to masking devices.
- Be prepared to reassess ongoing tinnitus, as new symptoms may develop. For example, tinnitus may precede other symptoms in Ménière's disease by months or even years.

- Depression in tinnitus has been severe enough to cause suicide. Make a thorough psychological assessment and consider a trial of antidepressants.
- Think of otosclerosis in younger patients (15–30) with persistent conductive deafness – especially if there is a family history. Early diagnosis is important.
- Progressive unilateral deafness with tinnitus could be caused by an acoustic neuroma. Exclude by referring for an MRI scan.

NOTES:

EYE

Acutely red and painful eye

Double vision

Eyelid problems

Flashes, floaters and transient visual disturbance

Gradual loss of vision

Itchy or irritating eyes or eyelids

Sudden loss of vision

ACUTELY RED AND PAINFUL EYE

The GP overview

This is a common reason for an urgent surgery appointment. If a visit request is made, try to negotiate consultation in surgery, where optimal examination conditions and equipment are to hand. Carefully examine to assess acuity, state of the cornea and pupillary reflexes.

Differential diagnosis

COMMON
- acute conjunctivitis (allergic or infective)
- acute iritis
- acute glaucoma
- keratitis/corneal ulcer
- corneal abrasion or superficial foreign body (FB)

OCCASIONAL
- episcleritis/scleritis
- keratoconjunctivitis sicca
- trauma: contusion and penetrating wound, burns (arc eye and chemical)
- orbital cellulitis

RARE
- carotico-cavernous fistula (rupture of carotid aneurysm)
- gout (urate deposits in conjunctiva or sclera)
- granulomatous disorders: TB, sarcoid, toxoplasmosis
- onchocerciasis (transmitted by *Simulium* black fly in Africa)
- tumour: primary eye tumour, invasion from nasopharyngeal tumour

Ready reckoner

	Conjunctivitis	Iritis	Glaucoma	Keratitis/ulcer	Abrasion/FB
Discharge	Yes	No	No	Possible	Possible
Visual disturbance	No	Yes	Yes	Possible	Possible
Circumcorneal injection	No	Yes	Possible	Possible	No
Poor pupil reflex	No	Yes	Yes	No	Possible
Hazy cornea	No	Possible	Yes	Possible	No

Possible investigations

In practice, the problem is either easily treated by the GP (e.g. conjunctivitis or foreign body) or usually requires urgent referral. The GP's role in investigating the painful red eye is therefore very limited.

- Swab of discharge for microbiology: very occasionally helpful in conjunctivitis not settling with usual treatment.
- Blood: raised WCC and ESR/CRP may support diagnosis of inflammatory disorders. Rheumatoid factor in suspected rheumatoid arthritis (RA); HLA-B27 usually positive in ankylosing spondylitis. The latter investigations would normally be performed at leisure rather than in the acute situation, when an underlying collagen disease is suspected (e.g. iritis).
- Intraocular pressure measurement is essential if acute glaucoma is suspected. Usually done by a specialist.

TOP TIPS

- If in serious doubt about the diagnosis, refer for urgent assessment – this is one scenario where a delay in treatment can have devastating consequences.
- Don't rely on the patient's subjective assessment of blurring of vision – check the visual acuity.
- Remember to evert the upper lid to check for a concealed foreign body.
- Review the patient 24–48 hours after removing a foreign body to ensure that the cornea has healed.

Red flags

- Never use mydriatics when examining the red eye: you may precipitate acute glaucoma.
- Bilateral red eye is usually caused by conjunctivitis. If unilateral, consider other causes.
- Failure to recognise herpetic corneal ulcer or acute glaucoma may lead to permanent visual loss. If in doubt, refer for urgent specialist opinion.
- Never instil steroid drops unless you are absolutely sure you are managing the problem correctly and have excluded herpetic ulceration.
- Take a careful history when dealing with foreign bodies. Any possibility of a high-speed impact (e.g. grinding metal) requires urgent specialist assessment to exclude intraocular foreign body.

NOTES:

DOUBLE VISION

The GP overview

Diplopia is nearly always binocular, with movement of one eye being limited for a number of possible reasons. Although relatively uncommon as a presenting symptom, the majority of causes are significant and therefore careful assessment is essential.

Differential diagnosis

COMMON
- physiological (focusing too near, or perceiving objects nearer than those focused on)
- intoxication: prescribed sedation, non-prescribed drugs, especially excess alcohol, opiates, benzodiazepines
- stroke
- mild head injury, causing temporary diplopia
- facial bone trauma – orbital and zygomatic fracture

OCCASIONAL
- mononeuropathy, e.g. diabetes, MS
- orbital disease (usually associated with pain and proptosis) and after surgery (scarring limiting globe movement)
- Guillain–Barré syndrome
- palsy of third, fourth or sixth cranial nerves due to intracranial space-occupying lesion (haemorrhage, tumour, aneurysm, abscess, cavernous sinus thrombosis)
- myasthenia gravis
- monocular diplopia: early cataract, irregularity of corneal surface, e.g. post trauma or inflammation

RARE
- ophthalmoplegic migraine
- Tolosa–Hunt syndrome: granulomatous or inflammatory process in anterior portion of cavernous sinus or superior orbital fissure
- pseudoparalysis of ocular muscles: dysthyroid disease; Duane's syndrome (congenital fibrosis of lateral rectus)
- orbital myositis
- pituitary exophthalmos

Ready reckoner

	Physiological	Intoxication	Stroke	Head injury	Facial bone trauma
History of trauma	No	No	No	Yes	Yes
Unequal pupils	No	No	Possible	Possible	No
Unilateral limb paresis	No	No	Possible	Possible	No
Impaired consciousness	No	Yes	Possible	Possible	No
Facial bone deformity	No	No	No	No	Yes

Possible investigations

LIKELY: none; FBC, ESR/CRP, lipid studies, urinalysis, fasting glucose or HbA1c.

POSSIBLE: TFT, X-rays, CT/MRI scan.

SMALL PRINT: edrophonium test, EMG, CSF studies, angiography.

- No investigation is indicated in primary care for the most common causes – referral is the likeliest course of action.
- FBC, ESR/CRP, lipid studies – if stroke suspected and admission not required. FBC and ESR/CRP will also provide evidence of inflammatory conditions.
- Urinalysis for glucose/fasting glucose or HbA1c – to investigate possible diabetes.
- TFT will reveal hyperthyroidism.
- Other investigations (and possibly some of the above) are likely to be carried out in secondary care: skull and facial bone X-rays in trauma cases; CT or MRI scan (head injury, stroke, MS, space-occupying lesion); specialist neurological investigations (edrophonium test, single-fibre EMG studies, CSF examination, angiography).

TOP TIPS

- Establish if the diplopia is binocular or not. Uniocular double vision has a much narrower differential diagnosis.
- Take time to clarify the symptom. Sometimes, patients complain of 'double vision' when they really mean blurring – and vice versa.
- The cover test is a reliable way to find out which eye is affected.
- Fourth cranial nerve palsy produces diplopia on looking downwards and inwards, often noticed when descending stairs. The patient may try to compensate by tilting the head – so-called ocular torticollis.

☑ Intoxication in conjunction with a head injury is commonly seen in custody medicine and A&E departments. Admission for neurological observation is strongly recommended.

☑ Diplopia of acute onset may well reflect serious pathology – refer for urgent assessment.

☑ Intermittent diplopia should not be dismissed too readily as insignificant – remember that myasthenia gravis and multiple sclerosis are possibilities.

NOTES:

EYELID PROBLEMS

The GP overview

Because of their close proximity to the eye, and their occasional cosmetic effect, eyelid problems can be disproportionately distressing to the patient. The differential diagnosis is wide – so the temptation to treat this presentation as a 'quickie' via a brief examination shouldn't distract from the need to take a careful history.

Differential diagnosis

COMMON
- stye
- blepharitis
- meibomian cyst
- xanthelasma
- blocked tear duct

OCCASIONAL
- periorbital oedema, e.g. orbital cellulitis, herpes zoster, angio-oedema, nephrotic syndrome, insect bite
- ectropion
- entropion (may be secondary trichiasis)
- eczema (seborrhoeic, allergic)
- ptosis (congenital, oculomotor nerve palsy, Horner's syndrome, myasthenia gravis, senile, myotonic dystrophy)
- muscular problems (myokymia, blepharospasm)

RARE
- malignant growth, e.g. basal cell carcinoma
- benign growths, e.g. papilloma, haemangioma
- dacrocystitis
- alopecia
- molluscum contagiosum
- lice

Ready reckoner

	Stye	Blepharitis	Meibomian cyst	Xanthelasma	Blocked tear duct
Painful	Yes	No	Possible	No	No
Long history	No	Possible	Possible	Yes	Possible
Visible swelling	Yes	No	Yes	Yes	No
Eye watering	No	No	No	No	Yes
Lids itchy	No	Yes	No	No	No

Possible investigations

LIKELY: lipid profile.

POSSIBLE: urinalysis, FBC, LFT.

SMALL PRINT: tests for ptosis, biopsy.

- Lipid profile: if xanthelasma, as may indicate hypercholesterolaemia.
- Urinalysis: proteinuria in nephrotic syndrome.
- FBC: WCC raised in infective process, e.g. cellulitis.
- LFT: hypoproteinaemia in nephrotic syndrome.
- Further tests for ptosis (usually in secondary care), e.g. CXR (Horner's), edrophonium test (myasthenia), blood sugar and brain scan (oculomotor palsy).
- Biopsy – if suspicion of malignancy.

TOP TIPS

- A meibomian cyst is often misdiagnosed – by patient and doctor – as a stye, particularly if it is infected.
- Entropion with secondary trichiasis may be overlooked as a cause of a recurring sore, watering eye, especially in the elderly.
- Myokymia – recurrent focal twitching of the orbicularis oculi – is harmless but may distress or alarm the patient.
- Many patients with xanthelasma will already have been 'noted' and so have had their cholesterol measured. Enquire about this before wasting resources on further unnecessary checks.

- Orbital cellulitis requires urgent inpatient treatment.
- Bilateral ptosis which deteriorates through the day may indicate myasthenia gravis.
- New onset of unilateral ptosis requires investigation – possible diagnoses range from diabetes to malignancy.
- Loss of the eyelashes is a poor prognostic sign in alopecia.
- Unilateral eyelash loss, with or without apparent blepharitis, may be a sign of an eyelid tumour.

NOTES:

FLASHES, FLOATERS AND TRANSIENT VISUAL DISTURBANCE

The GP overview

This symptom can be very difficult to fathom, not least because patients often find it nigh on impossible to describe exactly what they've experienced. Patience and a painstaking approach are essential – most of the clues are likely to be in the history rather than in the examination. This section does not cover double vision, gradual loss of vision or persistent sudden loss of vision, which are dealt with elsewhere.

Differential diagnosis

COMMON

- 'normal' floaters
- migraine
- posterior vitreous detachment
- amaurosis fugax
- retinal detachment

OCCASIONAL

- temporal arteritis
- vasovagals and orthostatic hypotension (commonly cause the symptom but rarely present with it)
- vitreous haemorrhage
- medication (e.g. transient blurred vision with anticholinergics, blue tinge to vision with sildenafil)
- poorly controlled diabetes
- TIA
- optic neuritis

RARE

- ▱ papilloedema
- ▱ trauma
- ▱ posterior uveitis
- ▱ seizures
- ▱ psychological

Ready reckoner

	Normal floaters	Migraine	Posterior vitreous detachment	Amaurosis fugax	Retinal detachment
Sudden onset	No	Yes	Yes	Yes	Yes
Blurred vision	No	Possible	No	Yes	Possible
Eye symptoms resolve in <1 hour	No	Yes	Possible	Yes	No
Flashing lights	No	Possible	Yes	No	Possible
'Curtain' effect	No	Possible	No	Yes	Possible

Possible investigations

The GP is highly unlikely to initiate any investigations in this situation – apart, perhaps, from a blood sugar or HbA1c to check for undiagnosed diabetes or an urgent ESR in suspected temporal arteritis. Otherwise, any investigations required would be arranged by the ophthalmologist or neurologist after urgent or routine referral, depending on the clinical picture.

TOP TIPS

- ▱ It is tempting to 'bounce' some of these cases to a local optician for assessment. Resist this approach – you may delay an important diagnosis and, besides, even a thorough examination is unlikely to provide anything like as much relevant information as a careful history.
- ▱ Some patients find it easier to 'draw' their visual disturbance than describe it.
- ▱ Floaters are a fairly common presentation – one of the key issues to establish is the duration of the symptom. The longer they have been present, the more you can be reassured that they are 'normal'.
- ▱ Remember that ocular migraine can occur without the 'usual' headache.

- [ ] A sudden onset of a shower of floaters is significant – especially if accompanied by flashing lights or blurred vision. Refer urgently to exclude a retinal detachment.
- [ ] Do not forget temporal arteritis as a cause of transient visual disturbance, especially in patients aged 50 or more. Treat with high-dose steroids on suspicion of this diagnosis – do not wait for the results of blood tests.
- [ ] Remember to check whether a young woman with migrainous visual disturbance is on the combined contraceptive pill and advise accordingly.
- [ ] Amaurosis fugax is a form of TIA and should be managed as such – apply your local 'TIA pathway'.

NOTES:

GRADUAL LOSS OF VISION

The GP overview

The four major causes of gradual blindness in the world are: cataract, onchocerciasis, vitamin A deficiency and trachoma. The latter three are very rare in the UK. Cataract occurs in 75% of over-65s, but only 20% of 45- to 65-year-olds. Most cases of gradual loss of vision encountered in primary care arrive via the optician, often with a letter outlining the problem and suggesting referral to an ophthalmologist.

Differential diagnosis

COMMON
- cataract
- chronic glaucoma
- diabetic and hypertensive retinopathy
- senile macular degeneration
- gradual inferior retinal detachment

OCCASIONAL
- choroidoretinitis
- optic neuritis (in MS)
- Paget's disease of the skull
- retinitis pigmentosa
- intraorbital or intracranial tumours

RARE
- syphilis
- cerebromacular degeneration
- toxic amblyopia (tobacco, methanol, arsenic, quinine, carbon bisulphide)
- choroidal melanoma
- Leber's hereditary optic atrophy

Ready reckoner

	Cataract	Glaucoma	Retinopathy	Macular degeneration	Retinal detachment
Unilateral visual loss	Possible	No	No	Possible	Yes
Pigment at macula	No	No	No	Yes	No
Exudate + haemorrhage	No	No	Yes	Yes	No
Fundus obscured	Yes	No	Possible	No	No
Disc cupped > 50%	No	Yes	No	No	No

Possible investigations

The only investigation the GP is likely to perform is a urinalysis and/or blood sugar or HbA1c for suspected diabetes. If glaucoma is a possibility, and the patient has not already seen the optician, then optician referral will provide information about fields and pressures. More obscure tests – such as posterior pole ultrasound and CT scan for retinal, or other, tumours; syphilis serology; skull X-ray for Paget's disease; and neurological investigations for MS – are rarely required and are inevitably arranged in secondary care.

TOP TIPS

- Opticians will tend to report cataracts in the elderly routinely. Referral for surgery is only required if the problem is significantly impairing the individual's normal activities.
- The presence of a cataract in relatively young patients is unusual and should prompt referral regardless of visual impairment – there may be a rare underlying metabolic cause.
- Remember that significant glaucoma or other causes of visual loss may render the individual unfit to drive.
- The elderly patient with a cataract whose vision is not improved considerably with the pinhole test probably has macular degeneration too, and so is unlikely to benefit much from cataract extraction.

- It can be very difficult to establish in an elderly person whether the problem really has been gradual in onset or whether the history is more sudden; if in doubt, refer urgently as the cause may be acute and remediable.
- Progressive early morning headache or proptosis with gradual loss of vision suggests a tumour. Refer urgently.
- Gradual or recurrent visual loss or blurring with other intermittent neurological symptoms, especially in younger patients, suggests the possibility of MS.

ITCHY OR IRRITATING EYES OR EYELIDS

The GP overview

This is a nuisance symptom which patients present with directly, or via their optician. It can be very difficult to ascertain whether the problem is arising from the eyelid or the eye itself. Often, the symptoms affect both and the causes overlap – which is why they're considered together here.

Differential diagnosis

COMMON
- allergic conjunctivitis (usually hay fever)
- infective conjunctivitis
- dry eyes
- blepharitis
- blocked tear duct

OCCASIONAL
- ectropion
- entropion
- eczema of the eyelids
- effect of contact lenses or solutions
- iatrogenic (oral or local medication)
- foreign body (though usually presents with pain and redness)

RARE
- pubic lice (can affect eyelashes)
- floppy eyelid syndrome (chronic conjunctivitis with lax eyelids in obese, middle-aged men)
- sebaceous gland carcinoma
- thyroid eye disease

Ready reckoner

	Allergic conjunctivitis	Infective conjunctivitis	Dry eyes	Blepharitis	Blocked tear duct
Bilateral	Yes	Possible	Yes	Yes	Possible
Eyes red	Yes	Yes	Possible	No	No
Eyelids red	Possible	No	No	Yes	No
Seasonal	Possible	No	No	No	No
Discharge	Yes	Yes	Possible	No	Yes

Possible investigations

LIKELY: none.

POSSIBLE: swab, Schirmer's test.

SMALL PRINT: TFT, thyroid autoantibodies, MRI orbits, biopsy.

- Swab: may be necessary in persistent discharge; essential in neonates who've had sticky eyes since birth.
- Schirmer's test: to assess for dry eye – may be performed by the optician.
- TFT, thyroid autoantibodies, MRI orbits – may be required in suspected thyroid eye disease.
- Biopsy: rarely, if sebaceous gland carcinoma suspected.

TOP TIPS

- Diagnosis can be difficult and an optician's input may be invaluable.
- Enquire about the use of OTC drops and their effect – this may give clues to the underlying problem. Sometimes, the drops themselves may be the cause.
- It can be easy to overlook entropion – ask the patient to squeeze the eyes shut, then suddenly open them, in which case a subtle entropion should be revealed.
- Bear in mind that patients with dry eyes sometimes paradoxically complain of a stringy discharge.

Red flags

- ◪ Remember that thyroid eye disease can present before biochemical dysfunction – if in doubt, refer.
- ◪ Do not overlook a foreign body as a possible cause, especially if the history is vague and the symptoms unilateral.
- ◪ Chlamydia and gonorrhoea must be excluded in the neonate with a sticky eye or eyes from birth.
- ◪ The rare sebaceous gland carcinoma causes blepharitis-type symptoms, but with localised inflammation and localised loss of lashes.

NOTES:

SUDDEN LOSS OF VISION

The GP overview

Sudden loss of vision is a genuine GP emergency. Most causes require an urgent ophthalmological opinion as there is little that the GP can do. This particular symptom is not often encountered in general practice – a prompt appointment or visit and a careful examination are necessary to assess the situation and exclude the causes not requiring urgent specialist treatment.

Differential diagnosis

COMMON
- acute glaucoma
- vitreous haemorrhage
- central retinal artery occlusion
- migraine
- CVA or TIA

OCCASIONAL
- central retinal vein occlusion
- retrobulbar (optic) neuritis
- retinal detachment
- temporal arteritis
- posterior uveitis

RARE
- hysteria
- cortical blindness (non-vascular)
- optic nerve injury
- quinine poisoning

Ready reckoner

	Acute glaucoma	Vitreous haemorrhage	Retinal artery occlusion	Migraine	TIA/CVA
Preceded by spots and flashing lights	No	Possible	No	Yes	Possible
Followed by headache	No	No	No	Yes	Possible
Painful eye	Yes	No	No	No	No
Absent red reflex	No	Yes	No	No	No
Affected pupil dilated and fixed	Yes	No	Yes	No	No

Possible investigations

In practice, there are none worth doing at the time, as the vast majority of cases will be referred urgently. Virtually all tests will therefore be arranged by the specialist, usually after the event, to look for underlying causes. Such investigations include the following.

- Screening for diabetes: undetected retinopathy may have preceded vitreous haemorrhage.
- FBC: PCV may be raised in central retinal vein occlusion.
- ESR: raised in temporal arteritis.
- Multiple microbiological investigations are needed for posterior uveitis.
- Posterior pole ultrasound may be useful in vitreous haemorrhage to identify treatable causes.
- CT scan only useful to investigate cerebral causes (CVA or cortical blindness).

TOP TIPS

- Acute visual disturbance is often difficult to diagnose accurately and very alarming for the patient. If in doubt, refer urgently, or, at the very least, review in a few hours.
- The patient's assessment of visual loss, and its severity, is highly subjective – if at all possible, test it with a Snellen chart.
- Always keep spare batteries handy for your ophthalmoscope!

- Don't forget that the visual disturbance may be the presenting symptom of some other pathology, such as hypertension, temporal arteritis or diabetes.
- Don't miss a heart murmur or carotid bruit. These may be present in retinal artery occlusion and TIA/CVA.
- A cherry red spot on the fovea is pathognomic of retinal artery occlusion.
- Never use mydriatics to aid examination at the bedside: these will cloud the clinical picture and may even precipitate acute glaucoma.

FACE

Facial pain

Facial rash

Facial swelling

Facial ulcers and blisters

FACIAL PAIN

The GP overview

Pain in the face may either be due to local disease of any of the major structures of the face, or conditions affecting the innervation. The latter can occur anywhere between the posterior fossa and the ends of the trigeminal nerve. A good examination is not difficult, and quicker than most as undressing is not usually required.

Differential diagnosis

COMMON
- maxillary/frontal sinusitis
- trigeminal neuralgia (TN)
- dental abscess
- temporomandibular joint (TMJ) dysfunction
- shingles (herpes zoster)

OCCASIONAL
- cluster headache (periodic migrainous neuralgia)
- temporal arteritis
- parotid: mumps, abscess and duct obstruction (stone/tumour)
- upper cervical spondylosis
- mandibular or maxillary osteitis or cyst
- cellulitis

RARE
- multiple sclerosis
- atypical facial pain (may be linked with depression)
- nasopharyngeal and lingual carcinoma
- posterior fossa tumours
- gummatous meningitis and tabes
- glaucoma and iritis

Ready reckoner

	Sinusitis	TN	Dental abscess	TMJ	Shingles
Fever and malaise	Possible	No	Possible	No	Possible
Lymphadenopathy	Possible	No	Yes	No	Yes
Pain worse on bending	Yes	No	Yes	No	No
Pain on tapping teeth	Possible	No	Yes	No	No
Lancinating pain	No	Yes	No	No	Possible

Possible investigations

LIKELY: none.

POSSIBLE: FBC, ESR/CRP, sinus X-ray.

SMALL PRINT: X-ray of TMJ, temporal artery biopsy, sialogram, CT/MRI scan.

- FBC: WCC and ESR/CRP raised in infection; ESR/CRP raised in temporal arteritis and tumour (ESR more useful than CRP in suspected temporal arteritis).
- X-rays: sinus X-ray of little help in acute sinusitis but may help in chronic pain to assess for possible chronic sinusitis or tumour; TMJ views and dental plain film for abscess likely to be arranged by dentist; parotid sialogram for stone/tumour.
- Temporal artery biopsy: may be necessary to clinch diagnosis of temporal arteritis.
- CT/MRI scan the only practical way to examine the posterior cranial fossa and Gasserian ganglion – a specialist investigation.

TOP TIPS

- Don't over-diagnose sinusitis – many URTIs will produce mild facial ache through a vacuum effect.
- Remember that shingles can produce pain before the rash – in the acute onset of unexplained unilateral facial pain, warn the patient to report back to the doctor should a blistering rash develop.
- Refer dental abscesses to a dentist without treating first, to ensure proper investigation, treatment and follow-up – and to encourage the patient to present to the correct agency in future.

- If no obvious cause is found for persistent facial pain, refer to exclude sinister pathology.
- Trigeminal neuralgia is usually idiopathic, but may have a serious underlying cause, especially if there is associated motor disturbance or other neurological symptoms or signs.
- Temporal arteritis is a clinical diagnosis. If suspected, treat immediately with high-dose steroids to prevent blindness. ESR is for retrospective confirmation only.
- If the eyeball is red and tender in frontal facial pain, consider glaucoma, iritis or orbital cellulitis. Refer urgently.
- Out-of-hours dental treatment can be very hard for patients to access in the UK. You may find yourself ethically obliged to provide some form of treatment, but be sure to give the advice (and document it) that the patient should contact their own dentist as soon as the dental surgery is open. Send a copy of your clinical notes to the dentist as you would any other clinician. You should never feel pressured to work outside your areas of competence, so don't hesitate to refer to the local hospital facio-maxillary team on call if you have any doubts about diagnosis or emergency management.

NOTES:

FACIAL RASH

The GP overview

Unlike the other 'skin' chapters in this book, this section is presented according to the rash's distribution. This is because it is a common presentation, one with a wide differential and one which causes the patient significant concern, largely because of the cosmetic impact. Occasionally, it can be caused by, or represent, significant pathology. Individual facial spots – such as basal cell carcinoma – aren't considered here.

Differential diagnosis

COMMON
- acne
- rosacea
- seborrhoeic eczema
- impetigo
- perioral dermatitis

OCCASIONAL
- chloasma
- sycosis barbae
- drug side effect – especially phototoxicity
- infection, e.g. herpes zoster and simplex, cellulitis, chickenpox, slapped cheek
- allergic eczema
- acne excoriée
- post inflammatory hypo- or hyperpigmentation
- pityriasis alba
- petechiae from coughing/vomiting/straining
- other generalised skin diseases, e.g. psoriasis, vitiligo

RARE
- Stevens–Johnson syndrome
- SLE
- mitral flush
- tuberous sclerosis
- lupus vulgaris
- sarcoidosis
- dermatomyositis

Ready reckoner

	Acne	Rosacea	Seborrhoeic eczema	Impetigo	Perioral dermatitis
Mainly around mouth	Possible	No	No	Possible	Yes
Rash elsewhere	Possible	No	Possible	Possible	No
Age >40	No	Yes	Possible	Possible	Possible
Papules and pustules	Yes	Yes	No	Possible	Yes
Rapid response to antibiotics	No	Yes	No	Yes	Yes

Possible investigations

LIKELY: none.

POSSIBLE: FBC, ESR, autoantibody screen, CPK.

SMALL PRINT: viral or bacterial swabs, skin biopsy, muscle biopsy.

- ◪ FBC: WCC raised in any infection; may be normochromic, normocytic anaemia in SLE.
- ◪ ESR, autoantibody screen: ESR likely to be raised in infection and SLE; autoantibodies may be positive in the latter.
- ◪ CPK: elevated in dermatomyositis.
- ◪ Viral or bacterial swabs: to help diagnosis in obscure cases or if secondary infection suspected.
- ◪ Skin biopsy; muscle biopsy: the former for suspected lupus vulgaris or sarcoidosis; the latter to confirm dermatomyositis.

TOP TIPS

- ◪ Do not underestimate the possible impact of a facial rash on a patient's life. The cosmetic effect may be devastating.
- ◪ A therapeutic trial of antibiotics in acne may take up to 3 months to take effect – ensure the patient is aware of this.
- ◪ Remember that impetigo may simply represent superinfection of an underlying skin problem, such as eczema, which will require treatment in its own right.
- ◪ Check on OTC medication usage. In particular, remember that hydrocortisone 1% cream is available over the counter – inappropriate use might aggravate rosacea and perioral dermatitis.
- ◪ Parents are sensitised to non blanching rashes. They can be reassured that such a rash restricted to the face (indeed, restricted to the entire distribution of the superior vena cava) is not due to meningitis.

- A complaint of dramatic facial 'sunburn' in the elderly may well represent a phototoxic reaction – check the drug history.
- Beware the acute onset of unilateral unexplained facial erythema with mild oedema, especially in an elderly patient. This may well be the start of cellulitis or herpes zoster.
- Warn patients with facial zoster or herpes simplex infection near the eye to report any ocular problems.
- Acne excoriée may be a marker of significant psychiatric pathology.

NOTES:

FACIAL SWELLING

The GP overview

This section looks at 'internal' causes of facial swelling rather than superficial skin conditions which are dealt with elsewhere (see p. 387). This problem is usually a major concern to the patient because of the disfigurement, which it is impossible to hide. The causal conditions are often very painful too.

Differential diagnosis

COMMON
- mumps (viral parotitis)
- angioneurotic oedema (allergy)
- dental abscess
- trauma (especially fractured zygoma)
- salivary gland stone

OCCASIONAL
- bacterial parotitis
- cellulitis (including orbital)
- masseteric hypertrophy (caused by bruxism)
- dental cyst
- myxoedema
- herpes zoster (may be swelling rather than blistering initially)

RARE
- parotid tumour
- maxillary or mandibular sarcoma
- Cushing's syndrome
- nasopharyngeal carcinoma
- Burkitt's lymphoma

Ready reckoner

	Mumps	Angioneurotic	Dental abscess	Trauma	Parotid stone
Bilateral	Yes	Yes	No	Possible	No
Swells when eating	No	No	No	No	Yes
Skin erythema	No	Yes	Possible	Possible	No
Tapping tooth painful	No	No	Yes	No	No
Fever	Yes	No	Possible	No	No

Possible investigations

LIKELY: facial X-ray (if trauma).

POSSIBLE: TFT (if patient looks myxoedematous).

SMALL PRINT: FBC, ESR/CRP, sialogram.

- Plain facial X-ray important in trauma (view may depend on site). Also may reveal rare cases of bony tumour.
- TFT, FBC, ESR/CRP: TFT will reveal hypothyroidism; WCC raised in infective process; ESR/CRP raised in infection and tumour.
- Parotid sialogram will show obstruction of duct (stone, tumour).

TOP TIPS

- New gruff voice with diffuse facial swelling should prompt investigation for likely hypothyroidism.
- Don't over-diagnose mumps in children: since the advent of MMR vaccination, this is becoming more uncommon; cervical adenitis is much more likely.
- Whenever possible, direct patients with dental problems directly to the dentist, who will be able to prescribe any necessary antibiotics and analgesics.

Red flags

- ☑ Painless, progressive facial swelling suggests tumour or dental cyst. Urgent oral surgical referral is indicated.
- ☑ Bloodstained nasal discharge in association with a unilateral facial swelling is an ominous sign suggesting malignancy.
- ☑ Severe angioedema may cause respiratory tract obstruction: treat vigorously as for anaphylactic shock.
- ☑ Orbital cellulitis requires urgent assessment and intravenous antibiotics.
- ☑ Parotid swelling with a facial palsy suggests parotid tumour with involvement of the facial nerve.
- ☑ Suspected herpes zoster in the ophthalmic division of the trigeminal nerve requires urgent antiviral treatment and ophthalmological referral.

FACIAL ULCERS AND BLISTERS

The GP overview

Facial ulcers and blisters present much earlier than similar lesions elsewhere on the body because of the cosmetic disfigurement. Smaller lesions, especially basal cell carcinomas, are often picked up coincidentally by the doctor when the patient attends for some unrelated matter. (NB: For rashes confined, or largely confined, to the face, see Facial rash, p. 153.)

Differential diagnosis

COMMON
- impetigo
- herpes simplex virus (HSV)
- herpes zoster
- basal cell carcinoma (BCC)
- keratoacanthoma

OCCASIONAL
- squamous cell carcinoma (SCC)
- ulcerating malignant melanoma and lentigo maligna (Hutchinson's freckle)
- drugs (e.g. barbiturates)
- acne excoriée
- ulcerating dental sinus

RARE
- dermatitis artefacta
- tuberculosis
- pemphigus
- *Actinomyces*
- primary syphilitic chancre or tertiary syphilitic gumma
- cutaneous leishmaniasis
- cancrum oris

Ready reckoner

	BCC	Herpes zoster	Keratoacanthoma	Impetigo	HSV
Feverish and unwell	No	Yes	No	No	Possible
Rapid development	No	Yes	Yes	Yes	Yes
Recurrent	Possible	No	No	Possible	Yes
Occurs in children	No	Possible	No	Yes	Yes
Multiple lesions	No	Yes	No	Yes	Yes

Possible investigations

Acute lesions very rarely require investigation; chronic lesions pose more of a diagnostic problem. In such cases, biopsy, or excision biopsy, is the gold standard test. Cytology after scraping the lesion with a scalpel blade may be helpful in diagnosing basal cell carcinoma. Syphilis serology may very rarely be useful if primary or tertiary syphilis is suspected.

TOP TIPS

- Remember that herpes simplex can occur on the face at sites other than the lip. The appearance of the lesions and their recurrent nature should provide the diagnosis.
- 'Rodent ulcer' is a kinder term than basal cell carcinoma, especially for small lesions, as it is less likely to arouse unnecessary anxiety. Nonetheless, impress upon the patient the importance of attending the appointment with the specialist.
- Patients with herpes zoster are at risk of a number of anxieties because of the existence of various 'old wives' tales' about shingles. Establish any fears and take time to explain the natural history of the condition, including the possibility of post-herpetic neuralgia.
- In children with recurrent impetigo, consider an underlying condition – particularly eczema.

- If in any doubt about the diagnosis, urgent dermatological referral for skin biopsy is indicated. Remember that chronic facial ulceration is rarely benign.
- Ulceration in a previously abnormally pigmented area of skin suggests advanced local malignancy.
- Beware attempting excision biopsy of facial lesions unless specially trained. Areas of cosmetic importance can be medico-legal minefields.
- Ask about foreign travel: leishmaniasis develops from the bite of a Mediterranean or South American sandfly.
- Beware of herpes zoster or simplex developing around the eye: significant complications may follow, so treat and follow up carefully and obtain an ophthalmological opinion if necessary.

NOTES:

GENERAL PHYSICAL

Abnormal gait in adults

Abnormal movements

Back pain

Crying baby

Delayed puberty

Episodic loss of consciousness

Excessive sweating

Failure to thrive

Falls with no loss of consciousness

The febrile child

Feeling tense and anxious

Flushing

Infertility

Itching

Jaundice in adults

Limp in a child

Numbness and paraesthesiae

Prolonged fever

Swollen glands

Thirst or dry mouth

Tiredness

Tremor

Weight gain

Weight loss

ABNORMAL GAIT IN ADULTS

The GP overview

Very few patients present with abnormal gait. It is more often noticed by the GP, while the patient's complaint is usually a manifestation of the gait (e.g. unsteadiness in Parkinson's disease) or of its cause (e.g. pain in arthritis). Congenital causes are not considered here as patients are most unlikely to present such problems to the GP.

Differential diagnosis

COMMON
- trauma (back and leg)
- osteoarthritis (OA) or other painful joint problem
- vestibular ataxia (vestibular neuritis, Ménière's disease, CVA)
- Parkinson's disease
- intermittent claudication (IC)

OCCASIONAL
- foot drop (peroneal nerve atrophy)
- multiple sclerosis
- spinal nerve root pain (especially L5 and S1)
- cauda equina lesions
- myasthenia gravis

RARE
- tabes dorsalis (syphilis)
- dystrophia myotonica
- motor neurone disease
- cerebellar ataxia
- hysteria

Ready reckoner

	Trauma	OA/other	Vestibular	Parkinson's	IC
Sudden onset	Yes	Possible	Yes	No	Possible
Painful unilateral limp	Yes	Yes	No	No	Yes
Worse with exercise	Yes	Yes	No	No	Yes
Shuffling gait	No	Possible	No	Yes	No
Staggering gait	No	No	Yes	No	No

Possible investigations

Most cases requiring tests will need referral to a specialist. The role of the GP in investigating these patients is therefore very limited.

LIKELY: none.

POSSIBLE: X-ray, FBC, ESR/CRP, RA factor, uric acid.

SMALL PRINT: scans, lumbar puncture, angiography.

- ◩ FBC, ESR/CRP, RA factor, uric acid: some forms of arthritis will result in an anaemia of chronic disorder. ESR/CRP may also be raised. Depending on the pattern of joint pain, RA factor and uric acid may provide useful information in the diagnosis of rheumatoid arthritis and gout.
- ◩ X-rays useful in bony trauma. Limited value in OA except to exclude other bony pathology.
- ◩ Syphilis serology: if tabes dorsalis suspected.
- ◩ If neurological signs of incoordination, consider CT/MRI scan and lumbar puncture – usually arranged by the specialist.
- ◩ Angiography: arranged by the vascular surgeon if surgery contemplated in claudication.

TOP TIPS

- ◩ Look up from the notes or computer as the patient walks in – otherwise you may miss a useful clue in the patient's gait.
- ◩ If the patient actually complains of problems walking, take your time in assessing the symptom – in particular, give the patient the opportunity to demonstrate the problem by walking him or her up and down the corridor.
- ◩ If the cause is not immediately apparent from the history, perform a careful neurological examination – this is a situation where there may be hard signs which contribute significantly to diagnosis.

☑ Vestibular neuritis usually settles within a few days. If patient remains ataxic, especially with persistent nystagmus, consider a central lesion and refer urgently.

☑ Numbness in both legs (saddle pattern) with back pain and incontinence suggests a cauda equina lesion. Admit urgently.

☑ If the patient is ataxic and has a past history of neurological symptoms, such as paraesthesia or optic neuritis, consider multiple sclerosis.

☑ Beware of labelling the patient as hysterical – apparently bizarre gaits may signify obscure but significant neurological pathology.

NOTES:

ABNORMAL MOVEMENTS

The GP overview

This is an infrequent cause for attendance – though the public is becoming increasingly aware of conditions such as restless legs syndrome (RLS) and Tourette's, and their treatments. Obvious generalised seizures and tremor are not considered in this chapter but are covered elsewhere.

Differential diagnosis

COMMON
- RLS
- myokymia (affecting orbicularis oculi muscles)
- drug induced – including choreoathetosis, dystonias, tardive dyskinesias and akathisia (drugs include l-dopa, tricyclic antidepressants, metoclopramide and antipsychotics)
- Tourette's
- simple partial seizures

OCCASIONAL
- anxiety/nervous tic (common, but rarely presented to the GP)
- muscle fasciculation (e.g. benign fasciculation, motor neurone disease)
- simple childhood tics (common, but infrequently presented)
- dystonias (e.g. writer's cramp, blepharospasm, spasmodic torticollis)
- period leg movements during sleep

RARE
- myoclonus
- chorea (Sydenham's, Huntington's)
- Wilson's disease
- hemiballismus (e.g. post stroke)
- hysterical

Ready reckoner

	RLS	Myokymia	Drug induced	Tourette's	Simple partial seizures
Worse at rest	Yes	Possible	No	No	No
Patient on medication	Possible	Possible	Yes	Possible	Possible
Whole limb affected	Yes	No	Possible	Possible	Possible
Other neurological signs	No	No	No	No	Possible
Childhood onset	No	No	Possible	Yes	Possible

Possible investigations

LIKELY: FBC, U&E, ferritin, B$_{12}$, folate, TFT, fasting glucose or HbA1c, calcium.

POSSIBLE: CT/MRI of brain or spinal cord, EEG, EMG, nerve conduction studies.

SMALL PRINT: other specialised tests (e.g. for myoclonus and Huntington's).

☑ FBC, ferritin: to assess for iron deficiency in RLS.

☑ U&E: renal failure is a potential cause of RLS and can be implicated in partial seizures.

☑ B$_{12}$, folate: deficiencies may cause or mimic RLS.

☑ TFT: hypothyroidism may cause RLS.

☑ Fasting glucose or HbA1c: diabetes may cause RLS or partial seizures.

☑ Calcium: hypocalcaemia may be implicated in seizures.

☑ CT/MRI of brain or spinal cord: may be required in investigation of fasciculation and seizures (usually arranged after specialist referral).

☑ EEG: for investigation of seizures.

☑ Other specialised tests: usually arranged by neurologist to explore the more obscure diagnoses such as Huntington's chorea and Wilson's disease.

TOP TIPS

☑ When faced with odd and otherwise inexplicable movements of recent onset in a patient, remember to take a drug history.

☑ Bear in mind that abnormal movements can be caused by a drug that the patient has been taking for some time (e.g. tardive dyskinesias).

☑ Patients with myokymia sometimes become disproportionately anxious about the symptom, imagining all sorts of possible neurological catastrophes – they may need a lot of reassurance.

☑ Childhood tics tend to be single; the patient with the much more significant Tourette's will probably have multiple tics.

☑ Drug-induced dystonias may cause odd posturing and require prompt treatment. The diagnosis is easily overlooked – antipsychotics are common culprits, so it is easy to erroneously attribute the dystonia to psychiatric pathology.

☑ Beware of the combination of personality changes and odd movements such as facial grimaces – this could be Huntington's chorea. Also, don't be misled by the lack of a positive family history – this background may have been concealed from the patient.

NOTES:

BACK PAIN

The GP overview

Ongoing backache is a familiar presentation to all GPs, and acute back pain is one of the most common reasons for an emergency appointment in primary care. The average GP can expect about 120 consultations for this problem each year. Eighty per cent of the Western population suffer back pain at some stage in their lives: it is the largest single cause of lost working hours among both manual and sedentary workers; in the former it is an important cause of disability. Remember that many non-orthopaedic causes of back pain lie in wait, so be systematic.

Differential diagnosis

COMMON
- mechanical (muscular) back pain
- prolapsed lumbar disc: nerve root pain
- spondylosis (exacerbation)
- pyelonephritis and renal stones
- pelvic infection

OCCASIONAL
- the spondoarthritides (e.g. ankylosing spondylitis, Reiter's syndrome)
- neoplastic disease of the spine (usually secondaries), myeloma
- duodenal ulcer/acute pancreatitis
- depression and anxiety states
- vertebral fracture (often compression fracture associated with osteoporosis)

RARE
- spinal stenosis
- osteomalacia
- aortic aneurysm
- pancreatic cancer
- spondylolisthesis
- osteomyelitis
- malingering

Ready reckoner

	Mechanical pain	Disc prolapse	Spondylosis	Pyelonephritis/ renal stones	Pelvic infection
Leg pain or numbness present	Possible	Yes	Possible	No	No
Unilateral symptoms	Possible	Yes	Possible	Yes	Possible
Depressed reflexes	No	Possible	Possible	No	No
Abdominal tenderness	No	No	No	Possible	Yes
Fever	No	No	No	Possible	Yes

Possible investigations

LIKELY: none.

POSSIBLE: urinalysis, MSU, FBC, ESR/CRP, plasma electrophoresis, blood calcium, PSA.

SMALL PRINT: lumbar spine X-ray, IVU, HLA-B27, CT or MRI scan, bone scan, investigations for GI cause, ultrasound, DXA scan.

- Urinalysis useful if UTI suspected: look for blood, pus and nitrite as markers of infection; confirm with MSU; blood alone suggests possible stone.
- ESR/CRP elevated in malignant and inflammatory disorders.
- FBC: Hb may be reduced in malignancy; a high WCC raises the possibility of osteomyelitis.
- Plasma electrophoresis: paraprotein band in myeloma.
- Blood calcium: elevated in myeloma and bony secondaries; reduced in osteomalacia.
- PSA: if disseminated prostate cancer suspected.
- Lumbar spine X-ray often not useful in mechanical pain. Consider if no resolution by 6 weeks to investigate possible underlying pathology. In younger patients, it may help diagnose sacroiliitis or spondylolisthesis; in older people, it is useful to check for vertebral collapse. Generally, if imaging is required, CT or MRI may be more helpful.
- Bone scan: will detect bony secondaries and bone infection.
- CT or MRI scan usually a specialist's request: good for spotting spinal stenosis, significant prolapsed disc and discrete bony lesions.
- Investigations for GI cause might include endoscopy (for DU), serum amylase (for pancreatitis) and CT scan (for carcinoma of pancreas).
- Ultrasound: for aortic aneurysm.
- IVU: for recurrent pyelonephritis and possible renal or ureteric stones.
- DEXA scan: may be required to confirm suspicion of osteoporosis.

TOP TIPS

- The vast majority are 'mechanical', and most of these improve regardless of treatment modality in 6–8 weeks; a positive and optimistic approach is important.
- Patients often expect an X-ray. Resist requests unless appropriate – and explain why. Even if the patient doesn't make this request, consider volunteering why you're not ordering an X-ray, as this can help maintain confidence in the doctor–patient relationship, especially if the symptoms take some time to settle.
- If the problem is recurrent, exclude significant pathology then explore the patient's concerns. In simple recurrent mechanical back pain, it is worth discussing preventive measures and educating the patient for self-management of future episodes.
- True malingering is not common, but back pain is favoured among malingerers because of its subjectivity. Beware of patients who apparently cannot straight-leg raise, yet have no problem sitting up on the couch, and patients who decline to sit down during the consultation.

- The traditional 'red flags' in back pain are thought to be of very limited use because of poor specificity and sensitivity. The only ones regarded as genuinely helpful are, for spinal fracture, older age, trauma, the presence of contusions or abrasions and steroid use, and, for spinal malignancy, a past history of cancer. Current consensus is that slavish adherence to red flags should be avoided and instead the overall clinical picture and progress assessed – although an ESR may be useful in ruling out significant disease.
- Bilateral sciatica, saddle anaesthesia and bowel and/or bladder dysfunction suggests central disc protrusion: this is a neurosurgical emergency.
- Consider prostatic cancer in men over 55 with atypical low back pain. Do a PR exam, together with PSA and bone assay.
- Back pain without any restriction of spinal movement, or which is not exacerbated by back movement, suggests that the source of the problem lies elsewhere – consider renal, aortic or gastrointestinal disease, or pelvic pathology in women.
- Tearing interscapular or lower pain in a known arteriopath suggests dissecting aortic aneurysm: admit straight away.

NOTES:

CRYING BABY

The GP overview

This is a very frequent reason for an out-of-hours call. A baby's cry is almost impossible for parents to ignore. When crying continues unabated in spite of all that parents can do to settle an infant, parental distress sets in and they will turn to you for an answer and a solution.

Differential diagnosis

COMMON
- normal
- colic
- constipation
- teething
- viral illness

OCCASIONAL
- otitis media or externa
- severe nappy rash and/or inflamed foreskin
- gastroenteritis
- UTI
- after immunisation
- respiratory distress – severe bronchiolitis, chest infection, croupy cough

RARE
- non-accidental injury
- mastoiditis
- meningitis, encephalitis
- septicaemia
- bowel obstruction including intussusception and strangulated hernia
- appendicitis
- osteomyelitis
- testicular torsion
- undiagnosed birth injury, e.g. fractured clavicle
- congenital disorders, e.g. Hirschprung's disease, pyloric stenosis

Ready reckoner

	Normal	Colic	Constipation	Teething	Viral illness
Reduced feeding	No	Possible	Possible	Possible	Yes
Drooling	No	No	No	Yes	Possible
Straining at stool	No	No	Yes	No	No
Fever	No	No	No	Possible	Yes
Tympanic abdomen	No	Possible	Possible	No	No

Possible investigations

LIKELY: none other than those performed after admission.

POSSIBLE: swab of any obvious discharge.

SMALL PRINT: see hospital investigations.

- Other than a swab for obvious discharge (e.g. in otitis externa), no investigations are appropriate in general practice – if no obvious cause is found and the baby continues to be distressed, admission for observation and investigation is mandatory.
- Secondary care investigations are likely to include urinalysis, MSU for bacteriology, bloods for FBC, ESR, glucose, U&E, and many others depending on the indication (e.g. CXR, AXR, lumbar puncture, blood gases).

TOP TIPS

- Babies cry on average for 1½ to 2 hours per day. Some normal babies cry more than this or for long periods for no apparent reason.
- Remain calm and sensitive. Parents of a crying baby are often distraught, and whatever your perception of the seriousness or not of the situation, make a thorough assessment and make sure the parents understand you are taking them seriously.
- Always explain your findings and advice clearly, and make sure the parents understand you. Write things down for them if necessary. Your patient depends completely on your communication skills.
- Remember the obvious – babies may cry because of tiredness, hunger, wind after feeds, boredom, and uncomfortably full nappies. Never assume that parenting skills are 100%, and do explore baby care issues that may seem to be too obvious to ask about.
- Babies may be unsettled and cry more than normal for a day or two after immunisation. If a baby is crying excessively for longer than 48 hours after immunisation, it is unsafe to diagnose immunisation as the cause without clinical assessment.
- Telephone advice calls may be handled with careful triage and advice alone, providing there is always a fall back plan for the parents to call back or seek further advice if things do not

settle rapidly. There is no substitute for a hands-on clinical assessment, and if in the slightest doubt, always see the baby as soon as possible.

▱ Observe in the most general way how a baby handles during examination. Irritability on handling is a very important general sign. Regardless of other examination findings, this alone can be a reason to refer for paediatric assessment.

▱ There is no clear physiological reason why babies should develop a fever during teething, but there is no doubt this happens in some babies, in spite of traditional medical teaching to the contrary. A fever is never high if due to teething alone. The fever of teething is usually very short-lived – less than 24 hours – while a fever caused by a viral infection can go on for several days.

▱ Babies cannot tell us what's wrong, but they can tell us *something's* wrong. If in any doubt about the diagnosis, seek a second opinion or a paediatric assessment. Always follow your sixth-sense, intuition or personal alarm bells. Thoughtful and experienced paediatricians will respect your feeling on this, so do not worry if you can't justify your referral on textbook clinical criteria.

Red flags

▱ Be aware of the possibility of non-accidental injury as a cause for the baby crying. If you detect unusual anxiety, or unusual emotional detachment from the calling parent, make sure you see the baby and examine it thoroughly.

▱ A baby that has been crying a lot and goes on to become lethargic (as opposed to a normal calm state) is probably very ill. Even if you are unsure of the diagnosis, follow your intuition and arrange a paediatric opinion.

▱ A constantly bulging fontanelle is always an indication for immediate paediatric referral.

▱ Be sure to observe and note the general muscular tone of a crying baby. Constant stiffness or floppiness are ominous signs and immediate referral is indicated.

NOTES:

DELAYED PUBERTY

The GP overview

Delayed puberty means delayed development of all the secondary sexual characteristics. It is a rare but serious symptom. In girls, it is usually presented as a delayed menarche (failure to menstruate by the age of 16), though it may present as failure to develop other secondary sexual characteristics from the age of 14. In boys, the defined age is 15. The following is a selection of the more important causes. (Remember that the subheadings Common, Occasional, Rare are relative – overall, this is a rare presenting symptom.)

Differential diagnosis

COMMON
- constitutional (50% of cases in boys, 16% of cases in girls)
- hyperthyroidism
- Turner's syndrome
- anorexia nervosa (1% of all girls in Western countries)
- hypothalamic gonadotrophin-releasing hormone (GnRH) deficiency (e.g. Noonan's and Kallmann's syndrome)

OCCASIONAL
- space-occupying hypothalamo-pituitary lesion (various types)
- chronic disease (e.g. diabetes, renal failure, cystic fibrosis, coeliac disease)
- hyperprolactinaemia
- adrenal disease: congenital adrenal hyperplasia and Cushing's disease
- drugs (e.g. thyroxine, chemotherapy (both sexes); androgens, anabolic steroids (females only))
- radiotherapy
- growth hormone deficiency

RARE
- other ovarian problems (e.g. pure dysgenesis, autoimmune disease)
- hypothyroidism if autoimmune (otherwise associated with early puberty)
- pure gonadal dysgenesis
- maldescent of the testes (rare nowadays: usually detected early)
- trauma, infection and granulomas of hypothalamus/pituitary

Ready reckoner

	Constitutional	Hyperthyroidism	Turner's	Anorexia	GnRH deficiency
Short stature	Possible	Possible	Yes	Possible	No
Anosmia	No	No	No	No	Possible
Otherwise well	Yes	Possible	Possible	No	Yes
Other physical signs	No	Possible	Yes	Possible	No
Family history	Possible	Possible	No	Possible	No

Possible investigations

Cases requiring investigation are likely to need referral to a paediatrician or endocrinologist. The role of the GP is therefore limited. A few basic tests might be arranged in primary care in probable constitutional cases, mainly to exclude underlying disease and 'reassure' patient, parents and doctor (e.g. urinalysis, FBC, U&E, TFT). More complex investigations in secondary care might include CT scanning (tumours), ultrasound of pelvis (to examine ovaries and search for non-palpable gonads), chromosomal analysis and various tests of endocrine function.

TOP TIPS

- Delayed puberty causes worry for parents and often misery for children, who may be teased or bullied by their adolescent peers. Take their concerns seriously from the outset.
- Remember to take a family history: constitutional delayed puberty often runs in families.
- The majority of children brought with 'delayed puberty' will be normal, with their parents either not recognising that secondary sexual characteristics are developing or not appreciating the age range which is normal for pubertal development.
- Distinguish between delayed puberty and primary amenorrhoea with otherwise normal pubertal development. The latter has different causes (e.g. vaginal atresia, cycle initiation defect and, very rarely, testicular feminisation).

- Although it accounts for 50% of male cases, do not diagnose constitutional delayed puberty in boys in the presence of a very small penis or anosmia – in these situations, an underlying disease is likely.
- More than 80% of cases in girls have a pathological cause, so investigation is the rule.
- Short stature, malaise and symptoms or signs of hypothyroidism suggest an underlying disorder of the hypothalamus and/or pituitary.

NOTES:

EPISODIC LOSS OF CONSCIOUSNESS

The GP overview

The terminology in this area can be very confusing with words like 'syncope' and 'faints' being used imprecisely. Episodic loss of consciousness can occur in any age group, though it tends to be commoner in the elderly. It is a frightening experience for the patient, and it demands thorough examination, investigation and a low threshold for referral. For the GP, the differential widens the older the patient – and cardiac causes should not be overlooked in the elderly.

Differential diagnosis

COMMON
- vasovagal attacks (faints)
- paroxysmal arrhythmia, e.g. Stokes–Adams attacks, sinus bradycardia, SVT
- epilepsy (various forms)
- hypoglycaemia
- orthostatic hypotension

OCCASIONAL
- cardiac structural lesion, e.g. aortic stenosis, hypertrophic obstructive cardiomyopathy, pulmonary stenosis
- micturition and cough syncope
- sleep apnoea
- Valsalva-induced syncope, e.g. weightlifting
- pseudoseizures

RARE
- narcolepsy
- carotid sinus syncope
- hyperventilation
- subclavian steal syndrome

Ready reckoner

	Vasovagal attack	Arrhythmia	Epilepsy	Hypoglycaemia	Orthostatic hypotension
Prodromal symptoms	Yes	No	Possible	Possible	Possible
Sweating	Yes	No	No	Yes	Possible
Trigger factors	Yes	No	Possible	Yes	Yes
Slow recovery	No	No	Yes	Yes	No
Abnormal resting ECG	No	Possible	No	No	No

Possible investigations

LIKELY: FBC; ECG (especially in elderly); if probable epilepsy, also EEG and CT scan.

POSSIBLE: glucometer, 24 h ECG.

SMALL PRINT: echocardiography, tilt-table testing.

- Glucometer 'on the scene' gives diagnosis of hypoglycaemia.
- FBC: anaemia will exacerbate any form of syncope and TIAs.
- Standard ECG may reveal signs of ischaemia and heart block; 24 h ECG more useful for definitive diagnosis of arrhythmia.
- CT scan and EEG essential if previously undiagnosed epilepsy suspected.
- Echocardiography: if structural cardiac problem suspected.
- Tilt-table testing: for unexplained syncope to assess susceptibility to vasovagal episodes.

TOP TIPS

- The key to diagnosis is an accurate history. This may not be available from the patient, so make a real effort to obtain an eyewitness account.
- In younger patients, the diagnosis is likely to lie between a vasovagal attack and a fit; in the middle-aged and elderly, the differential is much wider and will include, for example, arrhythmias and orthostatic hypotension.
- Episodic loss of consciousness is a symptom which merits diligent assessment. An accurate diagnosis has implications not only for the individual's health, but also for employment and driving.
- Remember that, with a vasovagal episode, patients remaining upright (e.g. sitting or in a crowd) may develop tonic–clonic movements which mimic a fit.
- Unlike in syncope or seizures, the eyes are usually closed in pseudoseizures.

- An eyewitness account that the patient looked as though he or she had died, together with marked facial flushing on recovery, is characteristic of Stokes–Adams attacks. These can be fatal, so early diagnosis is important.
- Discovery of an aortic stenotic murmur should prompt urgent referral. Severe aortic stenosis can cause sudden cardiac death.
- Red flags suggesting a possible cardiac cause include a family history of sudden cardiac death, syncope during exercise and an abnormal ECG.
- Syncope caused by neck pressure or head movement could be carotid sinus syncope – if recurrent, this will require a pacemaker.

NOTES:

EXCESSIVE SWEATING

The GP overview

Under normal conditions, 800 mL of water is lost daily as insensible loss, mostly in sweat. Excessive sweating can at least double this figure. As a symptom, it is normally part of a package of other problems – it is unusual for the patient to present with excessive sweating in isolation.

Differential diagnosis

COMMON

- menopause
- anxiety
- infections (common, acute)
- hypoglycaemia: may be reactive, i.e. non-diabetic
- hyperthyroidism

OCCASIONAL

- drugs: alcohol, tricyclic antidepressants, pilocarpine
- alcohol and drug withdrawal
- shock/syncope
- intense pain
- hyperhidrosis
- other infections, e.g. TB, HIV, endocarditis, brucellosis

RARE

- malignancy (e.g. lymphoma)
- organic nerve lesions: brain tumours, spinal cord injury (sweating is localised to dermatome involved)
- pachydermoperiostosis: localised to skin folds of forehead and extremities
- hyperpituitarism/acromegaly
- rare vasoactive tumours: phaeochromocytoma, carcinoid
- connective tissue disorders

Ready reckoner

	Menopause	Anxiety	Infection	Low glucose	Hyperthyroid
Short history	No	No	Yes	Yes	No
Vasoconstricted skin	No	Possible	Possible	Yes	Possible
Raised body temperature	No	No	Yes	No	No
Confusion	No	No	Possible	Possible	No
Systemically unwell	No	No	Yes	Yes	Yes

Possible investigations

LIKELY: FBC, ESR/CRP, TFT.

POSSIBLE: FSH/LH, LFT, glucose.

SMALL PRINT: autoimmune screen, CXR, tests for uncommon infections, 24-hour urinary catecholamines, CT/MRI scan.

- FBC/ESR/CRP: ESR/CRP and WCC raised in infection. Raised ESR/CRP and anaemia possible in lymphoma and other malignancies.
- TFTs: may reveal thyrotoxicosis as a cause of chronic sweating.
- Glucose: in reactive hypoglycaemia only useful at the time of the sweating.
- FSH/LH: helps if diagnosis of menopause in doubt.
- LFT: may reveal high alcohol intake.
- CXR might reveal occult infection (especially TB) or malignancy.
- Tests for uncommon infections, e.g. blood test for HIV, echocardiography for endocarditis.
- Autoimmune screen: may help in confirming diagnosis of connective tissue disease.
- 24 h urinary catecholamines traditionally used to look for phaeochromocytoma, but low specificity makes CT/MRI scan more useful.

TOP TIPS

- Length of history is very helpful – short-term sweating is likely to have an apparent, acute cause; if long-term, the diagnosis is more likely to be constitutional or anxiety; in the medium-term, the differential diagnosis is much wider.
- Anxiety rarely causes night sweats.
- Do not underestimate the potentially devastating effect of hyperhidrosis.

Red flags

- ☑ Lack of fever does not exclude infection. In some infections (e.g. TB, brucellosis) – and lymphoma – sweating can be out of phase with fever.
- ☑ If the problem is persistent, a full examination is advisable, paying attention to the lymph nodes, liver and spleen. If no cause is apparent, have a low threshold for investigations or referral, particularly if the patient is unwell or losing weight.
- ☑ Consider unusual infections in the recently returned traveller (e.g. TB, typhoid).
- ☑ Episodic skin flushing (especially provoked by alcohol) with diarrhoea and breathlessness is likely to be caused by anxiety – but don't forget carcinoid syndrome as a rare possibility.

NOTES:

FAILURE TO THRIVE

The GP overview

Failure to thrive is defined as the failure of a child to maintain the normal rate of growth for its age and gender. A logical and systematic approach is essential to navigate through the vast differential diagnosis list.

Differential diagnosis

There are very many causes of failure to thrive. To produce a workable list, we have given broad categories and emphasised within them the most common causes.

COMMON

- normal – the genetic components of height and weight kick in during the first 2 years, so babies of small parents may cross the centiles and appear to be 'dropping off'
- neglect (emotional and physical)
- feeding problems (inadequate or inappropriate feeding, physical causes, e.g. cleft palate)
- vomiting from any cause (gastro-oesophageal reflux common, other causes such as pyloric stenosis rarer)
- malabsorption – including cow's milk intolerance (lactose or cow's milk protein intolerance), coeliac disease

OCCASIONAL

- recurrent infections, e.g. UTI, frequent viral illnesses
- metabolic/endocrine causes, e.g. diabetes, hypo- and hyperthyroidism
- common chronic infection (UTI, gastroenteritis)
- syndromes, e.g. Turner's, Down's (though growth can follow centiles normally)
- intrauterine growth retardation
- premature delivery with complications
- toxicity during pregnancy, e.g. maternal smoking, alcohol, cocaine and amphetamines
- maternal medication or infection during pregnancy

RARE

- serious chronic disease, e.g. cerebral palsy, hepatic, cardiac or renal failure
- severe chronic asthma
- malignancy
- rare (in UK) chronic infection: TB, congenital HIV, parasites

- Munchausen's syndrome by proxy
- cystic fibrosis
- inborn errors of metabolism
- rare causes of infant feeding difficulties, e.g. hypotonia, micrognathia, Prader–Willi syndrome

Ready reckoner

	Normal	Neglect	Feeding problems	Vomiting	Malabsorption
Excessively hungry baby/child	No	Yes	Yes	Yes	Possible
Lethargic child	No	No	No	Possible	Possible
Diarrhoea	No	No	No	No	Yes
Fever	No	No	No	Possible	No
Associated parental psychosocial issues	No	Yes	Possible	No	No

Possible investigations

LIKELY: urinalysis, MSU, FBC, U&E, LFTs, thyroid function tests, coeliac screen, stool studies.

POSSIBLE: immunoglobulins.

SMALL PRINT: PPD skin test, radiological studies, sweat chloride test, growth hormone levels, HIV testing.

- Urinalysis and MSU to seek evidence of UTI.
- FBC may reveal both the effects of malnutrition (anaemia) and possible causes of failure to thrive, e.g. a raised white cell count indicating chronic infection.
- U&E and LFTs can both be markers of reduced metabolic function (reduced urea, creatinine and albumin, and reduced liver enzyme activity) or the signs of primary renal or hepatic disease.
- Thyroid function tests: essential and simple to detect over- or underactive thyroid.
- Coeliac screen and stool studies: for malabsorption (and look too for parasites, e.g. helminths or giardiasis).
- Immunoglobulins: different patterns and levels of different immunoglobulin classes are associated with a vast range of infective, autoimmune and neoplastic conditions.
- Purified protein derivative (PPD) skin test (for tuberculosis) is also known as the Mantoux test. A positive reaction to the injected tuberculin PPD may indicate current TB infection, or previous exposure.
- Radiological studies: bone age may be helpful to distinguish genetic short stature from constitutional delay of growth.

- Sweat chloride test is a reliable diagnostic test for cystic fibrosis, which affects 1 in 2500 infants.
- Growth hormone levels. Growth hormone deficiency affects about 1 in 3500 children.
- HIV testing if vertical transmission of HIV is suspected.

TOP TIPS

- Remember that 3% of normal infants fall below the third centile. Ask about height of other parent and grandparents in an otherwise healthy child. A constitutionally small child's growth will still follow the centile curves albeit from a low starting point.
- A third of children with psychosocial failure to thrive are developmentally delayed and have social and emotional problems.
- If parents are small, and there is no other sign of an underlying problem, it is safe to wait and observe the baby with regular weight measurements. The baby should return to running parallel with the centiles after the second year.

- A diagnosis of a non-organic cause of failure to thrive may be the earliest indication of a serious parent–child interaction dysfunction.
- Non-organically caused failure to thrive in the first year of life has an ominous prognosis. There is a high likelihood of ongoing child abuse in this group.
- If child abuse is suspected, refer to paediatrics urgently – by admission to hospital.
- The younger and more ill a child or baby is at presentation with failure to thrive, the more urgently assessment and action are required.
- A study has shown that half of cases of organic failure to thrive were also associated with a contributory psychosocial factor. Be alert to the fact that this can be a multifactorial condition.

NOTES:

FALLS WITH NO LOSS OF CONSCIOUSNESS

The GP overview

This is a common problem in the elderly and may represent an acute or chronic problem. A home visit is often necessary and can be very valuable, assisting diagnosis and management decisions.

NOTE: The term 'drop attacks' is inconsistently defined in the literature as 'falls with no loss of consciousness', 'falls with loss of consciousness' or may be regarded as a distinct diagnostic entity rather than a symptom. It is a term best left unused.

Differential diagnosis

COMMON
- orthostatic hypotension
- brainstem ischaemia (vertebrobasilar insufficiency)
- iatrogenic (e.g. phenothiazines, hypoglycaemics, tricyclics and hypotensives)
- postural instability (osteoarthritis, quadriceps weakness)
- any acute illness (e.g. sepsis, CVA)

OCCASIONAL
- lack of concentration (tripping over mats etc.)
- visual disturbance
- acute alcohol intoxication and chronic alcohol misuse
- Parkinson's disease
- cardiac arrhythmias
- any cause of vertigo (e.g. labyrinthitis, Ménière's disease) or non-specific dizziness (e.g. anaemia)

RARE
- hypothyroidism
- hydrocephalus
- third ventricular tumour
- diabetic autonomic neuropathy
- aortic stenosis
- painless ('silent') myocardial infarction

Ready reckoner

	Orthostatic hypotension	Vertebrobasilar insufficiency	Iatrogenic	Postural instability	Acute illness
Joint stiffness	No	No	No	Yes	No
On standing up	Yes	No	Possible	Possible	Yes
Confused	No	No	Possible	No	Possible
Polypharmacy	Possible	No	Possible	No	No
On turning head	No	Yes	Possible	No	Possible

Possible investigations

LIKELY: urinalysis, FBC.

POSSIBLE: TFT, LFT, ECG (or 24 h ECG).

SMALL PRINT: CT scan, echocardiography.

- Urinalysis for glucose may reveal underlying diabetes – a major cause of autonomic neuropathy – or evidence of UTI.
- FBC: anaemia will exacerbate any cause of postural hypotension, or may itself cause dizziness. Sepsis is suggested by a raised WCC. A high MCV may be a useful pointer to alcohol misuse or hypothyroidism.
- TFT: hypothyroidism is common in the elderly and develops insidiously.
- LFT: for evidence (γGT) of alcohol misuse.
- ECG or 24 h ECG is useful to identify an arrhythmia, conduction defect or MI.
- CT scanning (e.g. for tumours or hydrocephalus) or echocardiography (for aortic stenosis) may be arranged by the specialist after referral.

TOP TIPS

- Failure to observe the patient's gait may mean that significant diagnoses, such as Parkinson's disease, are missed.
- Recurrent falls in the elderly are often caused by a combination of factors, such as failing vision, poor lighting and trip hazards at home. A home assessment may give valuable clues.
- In the acute situation, management may depend more upon the ability of the patient to remain safely at home (e.g. social support) rather than the precise diagnosis.
- Don't underestimate the importance of what you prescribe in causing morbidity. Attempt to reduce polypharmacy and review therapy regularly.

- In dealing with this problem, don't forget to look for cause and effect: the aetiology of the falls and any significant injuries sustained.
- Sudden onset of falls in the previously well elderly patient is likely to represent acute pathology – have a low threshold for investigation or admission.
- Gradual onset of recurrent falls is often multifactorial in the elderly; in younger patients, specific underlying disease is more likely, so refer for investigation.
- Evidence of injury (e.g. bruises or fractures) and multiple attendance slips from A&E department indicate either a very frail, vulnerable elderly person or significant underlying illness.

NOTES:

THE FEBRILE CHILD

The GP overview

This symptom probably generates more GP advice calls and parental anxiety than any other. It is nearly always caused by an infection of some kind. The list of culprits is so vast that we have concentrated on the common and occasional ones more likely to be seen in general practice in the UK.

Differential diagnosis

COMMON

- non-specific viral URTI, e.g. colds, flu-type illness, pharyngitis, tracheitis
- gastroenteritis
- otitis media
- tonsillitis
- chest infection

OCCASIONAL

- urinary tract infection
- bronchiolitis
- croup
- common viral exanthems, e.g. chickenpox, roseola, hand, foot and mouth, fifth disease
- appendicitis
- cellulitis (especially orbital) and other significant skin infections, e.g. abscess, scalded skin
- glandular fever
- post-immunisation
- giardiasis

RARE

- meningitis/meningococcal septicaemia
- encephalitis
- hepatitis
- AIDS
- rare exanthems, e.g. measles, rubella
- mumps
- acute epiglottitis
- atypical infections, e.g. brucellosis, listeriosis, Lyme disease, cat scratch fever
- tuberculosis

- protozoal diseases, e.g. cryptosporidium, leishmaniasis, toxoplasmosis, malaria
- septic arthritis, osteomyelitis
- Kawasaki's disease

Ready reckoner

	URTI	Gastroenteritis	OM	Tonsillitis	Chest infection
Prominent neck nodes	Possible	No	Possible	Yes	Possible
Significant pain	No	Possible	Yes	Yes	Possible
Localising chest signs	No	No	No	No	Yes
Diarrhoea	Possible	Yes	Possible	Possible	Possible
Cough	Yes	No	Possible	No	Yes

Possible investigations

Usually none are necessary in practice. If a febrile child is ill enough to require investigation, the problem will usually be sufficiently urgent to need management by acute admission. Urinalysis, as a pointer to UTI (assuming obtaining a urine sample is feasible), is sometimes helpful in avoiding or facilitating admission. If possible, extend this to an MSU for bacteriological analysis.

TOP TIPS

- Many clinical markers (see Ready reckoner) are non-specific and are present in many different infections. It is often a matter of degree as to how likely they are a pointer to a specific pathology. For example, many infections cause mesenteric adenitis with abdominal pain, but the tenderness of appendicitis, for example, is usually far greater on examination. Respiratory rate is raised in all fevers, but a chest problem will increase it further along with the presence of chest signs. A good policy is to be as thorough as possible in an examination so as to be able to cross-reference the maximum clinical information.
- Remember that parents will be worried about their child, and no matter how simple the management of this common problem appears to you, to the parent it may be the harbinger of a serious illness. Practise a calm and polite demeanour, empathy and sensitivity.
- In telephone advice calls, always do three things: first, check that the parent is satisfied with your advice; second, put a robust safety net/plan B in place with easily identifiable guidelines for the parent, e.g. 'if by X hours Y has not happened, then call back'; third, record your clinical assessment and the last two points in detail.
- If in doubt, always see a child in person. Be sensitive to your intuition. If something nags

you after an advice call, ring back and arrange a consultation. You will never look stupid for doing this – only careful.

- Remember to follow up children in whom you've diagnosed UTI according to NICE guidelines, which recommend further investigation, varying according to the age of the child.

- It is very easy to print computerised clinical notes immediately after writing them. Handing a consultation note to a parent can be invaluable to the parent (and the clinician) if the child is seen later on out of hours, when clinical records are often unavailable. The baseline findings from earlier in the day can be priceless information in the dark hours later on.

- Spend time explaining the nature of fever and that the key issue is the cause of the fever rather than the fever itself – many parents are 'fever phobic'.

- It's often more important to be able to distinguish between 'well' and 'ill' babies and children than it is to make a clever, precise diagnosis – the NICE 'traffic light' guidance may help.

- It's easy to be tempted into complacency in the telephone or consultation management of this problem – fever is just so common. Never forget that uncommon very serious illnesses may all begin with a fever. Always be diligent and systematic in assessment, no matter how busy your winter on-call day is turning out to be.

Red flags

- Dehydration can kill a baby quickly. Ensure you have satisfied yourself about the state of hydration of a child. The colour and quantity of urine passed, or frequency of nappy changes are useful practical guides, together with the general 'look' of the child and the capillary refill time.

- A febrile baby or child who is floppy or drowsy should be admitted immediately.

- Be suspicious of the irritable and inconsolable infant. Even without other hard evidence, suspect a serious problem and arrange urgent paediatric assessment.

- The petechial rash of meningococcal septicaemia is a late phenomenon. Do not be reassured by its absence. Its presence should prompt a 999 call and administration of immediate parenteral antibiotics according to local protocols.

- In most cases, the height of a fever is no guide to the severity of the illness – the exception being babies, where a temperature of 38°C or more in those under 3 months is seen as a 'red' and one of 39°C or more in those between 3 and 6 months is viewed as 'amber' according to NICE.

NOTES:

FEELING TENSE AND ANXIOUS

The GP overview

The patient complaining of feeling tense and anxious may induce similar feelings in the GP – because there are many possible underlying and contributory causes, the consultation may be lengthy, and the patient may well present in a crisis. A calm, methodical approach, possibly stretching over more than one consultation, will pay dividends.

Differential diagnosis

COMMON
- ☑ life events (may be underlying 'anxious personality')
- ☑ pre-menstrual tension
- ☑ generalised anxiety disorder
- ☑ panic disorder
- ☑ depression

OCCASIONAL
- ☑ obsessive–compulsive disorder
- ☑ phobias
- ☑ drug side effect (for example, in the early stages of SSRI treatment)
- ☑ hyperthyroidism
- ☑ drug/alcohol use or withdrawal
- ☑ somatisation disorder
- ☑ post-traumatic stress disorder

RARE
- ☑ psychotic illness
- ☑ any cause of palpitations (may be 'misinterpreted' by the patient or others as anxiety)
- ☑ organic brain disease, e.g. tumour

Ready reckoner

	Life events	PMT	GAD	Panic disorder	Depression
Clear causative event	Yes	No	No	No	Possible
Related to menstrual cycle in women	No	Yes	Possible	No	Possible
Persistent low mood	Possible	No	No	No	Yes
Feeling of tension is short-lived	Possible	Possible	No	Yes	Possible
Sleep disturbed	Yes	Possible	Possible	No	Yes

Possible investigations

It would be very unusual for the GP to require any investigations when dealing with this symptom. Thyroid function tests would be indicated in suspected hyperthyroidism, and a blood screen, to include LFT, if alcohol was thought to be playing a significant part. Investigations in the rare event of suspected organic brain disease would usually be left to the specialist.

TOP TIPS

☑ It is tempting to lump many of these scenarios under a catch-all label of 'tension' or 'anxiety'. But attempts at making a more precise diagnosis are worthwhile, as this may significantly alter the management.

☑ Do not overlook an alcohol or drug history: abuse or withdrawal may be the cause of the symptoms, or a significant contributor.

☑ It may be worthwhile carefully reviewing the patient's old records to establish patterns of symptoms or attendance, and to check previous response to treatment.

☑ Whenever possible, life events should not be 'medicalised' – otherwise this may, in the future, encourage re-attendance and foster dependence on treatment.

☑ Apparent pre-menstrual tension may be a sign of some other underlying disorder – the patient may be suffering generalised anxiety disorder, for example, but may tend to focus on the pre-menstrual phase, when the symptoms are at their worst.

☑ Do not accept a self-diagnosis of 'panic attacks' at face value – the patient may actually mean any one of a number of possible symptoms.

- If the underlying diagnosis turns out to be depression, assess for any suicidal ideas or intent.
- Check for any psychotic features – anxiety can occasionally be a presenting feature of serious psychotic illness.
- New onset of tension or anxiety without any obvious explanation – especially in the context of personality change, neurological features or new headaches – could, rarely, reflect organic brain disease.
- It's important to make diagnoses such as somatisation disorder when appropriate – otherwise the patient may suffer years of unnecessary tests and treatment.

NOTES:

FLUSHING

The GP overview

This symptom presents more often in women than in men, not only because of its cosmetic importance, but also because the menopause accounts for the vast majority of presentations. It is different from emotional blushing in its context, severity, duration and extent.

Differential diagnosis

COMMON
- menopause
- chronic alcohol misuse
- rosacea
- iatrogenic (e.g. calcium antagonists)
- anxiety

OCCASIONAL
- polycythaemia rubra vera
- hyperthyroidism
- drug/alcohol interaction: metronidazole, disulfiram
- mitral valve disease (malar flush)
- hyperglycaemia and hypoglycaemia
- epilepsy (aura)

RARE
- carcinoid tumour
- phaeochromocytoma
- Zollinger–Ellison syndrome
- systemic mastocytosis
- ACTH-secreting bronchogenic carcinoma and Cushing's syndrome

Ready reckoner

	Menopause	Alcohol	Rosacea	Iatrogenic	Anxiety
Continuous	No	Possible	Possible	Possible	No
Weight loss	No	Possible	No	No	Possible
Facial papules	No	No	Yes	No	No
Tremor	No	Possible	No	No	Yes
Long history	Possible	Yes	Possible	No	Possible

Possible investigations

LIKELY: none.

POSSIBLE: FBC, LFT, TFT, blood sugar.

SMALL PRINT: echocardiogram, EEG, urinary 5HIAA and VMA, gastrin level, further specialised endocrine tests.

- ☑ FBC: raised haemoglobin and PCV in polycythaemia (may also be elevated platelets and WCC), raised MCV in chronic alcohol misuse.
- ☑ Biochemistry: LFT and γGT abnormal in alcohol misuse. TFT will reveal hyperthyroidism.
- ☑ Blood sugar: to reveal hypo- or hyperglycaemia.
- ☑ FSH/LH of limited use as does not correlate well with symptoms (useful only if premature menopause suspected).
- ☑ Echocardiography: if mitral stenosis suspected.
- ☑ EEG: for possible epilepsy.
- ☑ Specialist tests might include urinary 5HIAA (carcinoid) and VMA (phaeochromocytoma), gastrin level (Zollinger–Ellison syndrome) and further endocrine tests (e.g. for Cushing's syndrome).

TOP TIPS

- ☑ Most women complaining of flushing will suspect the cause is the menopause. Address this possibility in the consultation, especially in young women fearing 'an early change'.
- ☑ A constantly flushed face in older men is likely to be due to alcohol, polycythaemia or rosacea.
- ☑ Anxiety is likely if the circumstances fit – but bear in mind that hyperthyroidism can produce a very similar clinical picture.
- ☑ It can be difficult to distinguish anxiety from menopausal symptoms in a woman of menopausal age. Flushes with sweats waking the woman at night are more likely to be caused by the menopause – but a trial of treatment is the acid test (though beware of an initial placebo response).

- Diarrhoea and dyspnoea with flushing after alcohol, food and exercise suggest possible carcinoid syndrome.
- Flushing followed by an episode of altered consciousness points to a significant cause, such as recurrent hypoglycaemia or epilepsy.
- Do not be tempted to write this symptom off as the hot flushes of emotional blushing. While common, this problem is unlikely to present in daily practice.
- Recent onset of severe flushing which is not obviously menopausal or anxiety may have a significant cause, especially if the patient has other symptoms. Have a low threshold for investigations or referral in such cases.

NOTES:

INFERTILITY

The GP overview

About 80% of couples conceive within the first year of trying, and a further 5–10% in the second. Infertility is defined as a failure to conceive after 2 years of regular intercourse. However, depending on the circumstances, it may be appropriate for the GP to intervene before this arbitrary 2-year cut-off. Management is likely to be dictated by prevailing national and local guidelines and protocols.

Differential diagnosis

COMMON
- unexplained (27%)
- defective sperm (24% – may be various underlying causes)
- anovulatory cycles/defective ovulation (21%)
- fallopian tube blockage (14%)
- endometriosis (6%)

OCCASIONAL
- hostile cervical mucus
- PCOS
- other causes of amenorrhoea or hypomenorrhoea (see Absent periods, p. 374)
- uterine fibroids, polyp
- cervical problems: inflammation, polyps, stenosis
- systemic illness, e.g. anaemia, thyroid disorders

RARE
- congenital uterine, vaginal, fallopian or ovarian malformation or absence
- sexual dysfunction
- adrenocortical tumours
- chromosomal abnormalities: Turner's syndrome (XO), super-female (XXX)
- endometrial tuberculosis

Ready reckoner

	Unexplained	Defective sperm	Anovulation/ defective ovulation	Tubal blockage	Endometriosis
Dysmenorrhoea	No	No	No	Possible	Yes
History of STD	No	Possible	No	Yes	No
Menorrhagia	No	No	Possible	Possible	Possible
Abnormal pelvic examination	No	No	No	Possible	Possible
Regular cycle	Yes	Yes	Possible	Yes	Yes

Possible investigations

NOTE: amenorrhoea will need investigation in its own right – see Absent periods, p. 374. The degree of investigation undertaken for infertility will depend very much on the particular situation and local guidelines.

LIKELY: semen analysis, serum progesterone 7 days before anticipated onset of period.

POSSIBLE: if menstrual irregularity/amenorrhoea/unwell – FBC, FSH, LH, prolactin, TFT, U&E, testosterone. In secondary care: ovarian/uterine ultrasound.

SMALL PRINT: laparoscopy and dye, hysterosalpingogram, post-coital test. In the male: further investigation of sperm problems, e.g. FSH, LH, testosterone, testicular ultrasound.

- Semen analysis: may need repeating if first test sub-optimal.
- Serum progesterone 7 days before anticipated onset of period: to check for ovulation.
- FBC, FSH, LH, prolactin, TFT, U&E, testosterone: to check for underlying pathology if female is unwell or has menstrual problems.
- Ovarian and uterine ultrasound: to exclude structural abnormalities. Can be extended to visualise ovarian follicle development and ovulation.
- Laparoscopy and dye, hysterosalpingogram: to check for tubal patency.
- Post-coital test: cervical mucus sampled 12 hours post-coitally is examined under high-power microscope. More than 10 motile sperm per high-power field implies satisfactory coitus, adequate sperm and antibody-free cervical mucus.
- Male FSH, LH and testosterone: to check for endocrine causes of sperm production failure.
- Testicular ultrasound: if anatomical abnormalities found on examination, e.g. varicocoele.

TOP TIPS

- Adopt an optimistic approach whenever possible. A surprising number of couples conceive successfully as soon as preliminary investigations are initiated!
- Don't overlook health promotion opportunities – especially female rubella status and advice about taking folic acid.

- Ensure you treat the couple rather than the individuals. Infertility management requires much cooperation and motivation.
- In primary care, hormone tests (other than progesterone) are not necessary if the periods are normal.

- Infertility will only very rarely be the presenting symptom of serious pathology. However, there are circumstances where it is important to act promptly in terms of investigation or referral, such as:
  - if the female
    - is over the age of 35
    - has amenorrhoea
    - has a history of previous pelvic surgery or PID
    - has any abnormality on pelvic examination
  - or if the male
    - has a history of urogenital problems or STD
    - has a varicocoele.

NOTES:

ITCHING

The GP overview

Itching is the commonest presenting dermatological symptom. It is frequently distressing, and may interfere with the patient's quality of life – for example, by preventing normal sleep. Therefore, it should be taken seriously. A good history alone will reveal the diagnosis in the majority of cases. The remainder will yield to thorough examination and investigation. Dermatological referral need only be a last resort to achieve diagnosis.

Differential diagnosis

COMMON
- contact allergy (contact dermatitis)
- scabies (and other pediculoses)
- atopic eczema
- pityriasis rosea
- psoriasis

OCCASIONAL
- urticaria (e.g. food or drug allergy)
- jaundice of any cause
- iron deficiency anaemia
- endocrine: diabetes mellitus, hypo- and hyperthyroidism
- renal failure (uraemia)
- lichen planus
- prickly heat

RARE
- herpes gestationis
- dermatitis herpetiformis
- psychogenic (includes dermatitis artefacta)
- leukaemia and myeloproliferative disorders
- simple pruritus: no other cause found
- drug side effect (with or without rash)

Ready reckoner

	Contact allergy	Scabies	Atopic eczema	Pityriasis rosea	Psoriasis
History of chemical exposure	Yes	No	Possible	No	No
Widespread itch	Possible	Yes	Possible	Yes	No
Worse at night	No	Yes	Possible	No	No
Mainly on flexures	No	No	Yes	No	No
Mainly on extensor surfaces	Possible	No	No	No	Yes

Possible investigations

LIKELY: none.

POSSIBLE: urinalysis, blood glucose or HbA1c, FBC, ESR, U&E, LFT, TFT.

SMALL PRINT: none.

- Urine: dipstick for glycosuria (blood glucose or HbA1c if positive).
- FBC: will reveal iron-deficiency anaemia and polycythaemia; eosinophil count may be raised in allergic conditions; WCC may be very high in leukaemia; ESR may be elevated in lymphoma.
- U&E: will reveal uraemia.
- LFT: deranged liver enzymes and raised bilirubin in liver disease.
- TFT: both hypo- and hyperthyroidism can lead to skin changes which cause itching.

TOP TIPS

- An itchy, unidentifiable rash which is worse at night is likely to be scabies, particularly if any contacts are affected.
- Warn the patient that scabies treatment may take a week or two fully to relieve symptoms – otherwise, the patient may apply the treatment repeatedly, causing a chemical irritation and diagnostic confusion.
- The books usually state that psoriasis doesn't itch – but it certainly can, so don't let this symptom put you off the diagnosis.
- It is usually very difficult to identify the allergen in a single episode of urticaria. Tell the patient to keep a note of foods or medicines just ingested so that, in the event of recurrence, the culprit can be identified.

- If no obvious cause, always examine the abdomen and lymph nodes: do not miss lymphadenopathy, or enlarged liver, spleen or kidneys.
- Don't be tempted not to examine the itchy, malodorous self-neglected patient: poor personal hygiene may deceptively mask some other identifiable underlying cause.
- Beware of apparently florid eczema appearing for the first time in an elderly patient – this may be a manifestation of serious underlying pathology.
- Don't forget iatrogenic causes – enquire about any drugs recently prescribed.

NOTES:

JAUNDICE IN ADULTS

The GP overview

Patients rarely present with the complaint of 'turning yellow'; more often – though still infrequently – the GP notices jaundice during an examination of the patient. A systematic clinical assessment together with relevant laboratory investigations will help pinpoint the cause.

Differential diagnosis

COMMON
- gallstones in common bile duct
- viral hepatitis (e.g. glandular fever, hepatitis A, B, C)
- carcinoma of head of pancreas
- hepatic carcinoma (usually metastases)
- alcoholic cirrhosis

OCCASIONAL
- alcoholic hepatitis
- primary biliary cirrhosis
- drugs: chlorpromazine, isoniazid, anabolic steroids, methyldopa, paracetamol overdose
- haemolytic anaemia (many causes, such as autoimmune, malaria, drugs)
- venous congestion: cardiac failure, constrictive pericarditis
- cholangitis (and stricture in common bile duct afterwards)
- pancreatitis

RARE
- carcinoma of bile duct
- leptospirosis
- Rotor, Dubin–Johnson and Mirizzi syndromes
- cholestasis or fatty liver of pregnancy
- genetic: Gilbert's syndrome, Wilson's disease, α_1-antitrypsin deficiency, galactosaemia, glycogen storage diseases, haemochromatosis
- amyloidosis

Ready reckoner

	Gallstones	Hepatitis	Carcinoma of pancreas	Metastases	Alcohol cirrhosis
Fever	Possible	Yes	No	No	No
Colicky RUQ pain	Yes	No	No	No	No
Rapid weight loss	No	Possible	Yes	Yes	No
Pale stools/dark urine	Yes	Possible	Yes	No	No
Epigastric mass	No	No	Yes	Possible	No

Possible investigations

LIKELY: urinalysis, FBC, LFT, hepatitis serology.

POSSIBLE: ultrasound, antimitochondrial antibody.

SMALL PRINT: serum amylase, secondary care tests (e.g. ERCP, liver biopsy).

- Urinalysis: if bilirubin is present in the urine, the jaundice is cholestatic. If present with urobilinogen, it is hepatocellular. If not, it is obstructive.
- LFT: bilirubin very high in biliary obstruction. AST and ALT raised in hepatic causes. Alkaline phosphatase rises moderately in hepatic causes and markedly in biliary obstruction and primary biliary cirrhosis.
- FBC: anaemia in chronic illness. Raised WCC in hepatitis. May be macrocytosis, reticulocytosis and other red cell abnormalities in haemolytic anaemia. MCV raised by alcohol.
- Hepatitis serology: may reveal cause of viral hepatitis.
- Serum amylase: raised in pancreatitis.
- Antimitochondrial antibody test: positive in over 95% of patients with primary biliary cirrhosis.
- Ultrasound useful to assess liver, pancreas and gall bladder: may reveal stones, primary tumours and metastases.
- Referral may result in various other specialised tests including ERCP and liver biopsy, to establish the underlying cause.

TOP TIPS

- Remember to look at the patient: if significant jaundice is present it will probably strike you at first glance.
- In younger patients, the diagnosis is likely to be viral hepatitis. In older age groups, the differential is much wider.
- Don't forget iatrogenic causes. Remember too that the presence of jaundice implies liver dysfunction, so take great care if prescribing any medication.
- If the patient is well, with no pain and fever, it is reasonable to arrange initial investigations

– especially LFT – and arrange for review in a day or two. Most other cases will require admission.

☑ Remember to ask about foreign travel, contact with travellers, drug misuse and sexual history if necessary in the suddenly jaundiced febrile patient.

☑ Painless progressive jaundice suggests carcinoma of pancreas. Refer urgently.

☑ An enlarged, knobbly, hard liver is nearly always caused by metastases.

☑ Beware of restlessness, poor concentration and drowsiness. These suggest fulminant hepatic failure.

NOTES:

LIMP IN A CHILD

The GP overview

This is an infrequent but alarming presentation, as it may herald significant pathology and may be difficult to manage properly in an uncooperative toddler. Assessment should be methodical and patient, and follow-up arranged unless the diagnosis is obvious at the outset.

Differential diagnosis

COMMON
- trauma, including foreign body in foot (especially toddlers)
- irritable hip (transient synovitis)
- acute viral infection with arthralgia
- pauciarticular juvenile chronic arthritis (JCA: 1 in 1000)
- slipped femoral epiphysis (usually over 10 years old)

OCCASIONAL
- Perthes's disease (1 in 2000 between 4 and 10 years old)
- septic arthritis
- idiopathic scoliosis
- congenital dislocation of the hip (5–10 per 1000)
- acute lower abdominal pain – especially appendicitis
- unequal leg length
- neurological, e.g. cerebral palsy

RARE
- acute osteomyelitis
- rheumatic fever
- autoimmune disorders (e.g. SLE, dermatomyositis)
- rickets
- genuine juvenile rheumatoid arthritis
- malignancy affecting bone
- Duchenne's muscular dystrophy

Ready reckoner

	Trauma	Irritable hip	Viral infection	JCA	Slipped epiphysis
Fever	No	Possible	Yes	Possible	No
Sudden onset	Yes	Possible	Possible	No	Yes
Stiff in early morning	No	No	No	Yes	No
Usually over 10 years old	No	No	No	No	Yes
Many joints affected	No	No	Yes	Possible	No

Possible investigations

LIKELY: FBC, ESR/CRP, X-ray.

POSSIBLE: autoimmune screen.

SMALL PRINT: calcium, phosphate, alkaline phosphatase, creatine kinase, ASO titre, blood culture.

- FBC and ESR/CRP: WCC and ESR/CRP elevated in an underlying inflammatory or infective cause.
- Hip X-ray: may reveal fracture, slipped femoral epiphysis, congenital dislocation, Perthes's and other significant disorders – but may be normal in the presence of serious pathology.
- Rheumatoid factor and autoimmune screen may be helpful if a connective tissue disorder is suspected.
- Serum calcium, phosphate and alkaline phosphatase: calcium and phosphate low, alkaline phosphatase high in rickets.
- Creatine kinase: markedly elevated in muscular dystrophy.
- ASO titre is raised in 80% of cases of rheumatic fever.
- In hospital, blood culture may identify the infecting organism in osteomyelitis and septic arthritis.

TOP TIPS

- Never forget to examine the soles of the feet and between the toes for obvious and potentially simple to treat, non-serious causes of limp.
- It's worth investing some time gaining the child's confidence – this will enable you to make a proper assessment and feel positive about your management.
- Parents may try to rationalise the symptom by recalling a recent minor episode of trauma which is likely to be purely coincidental.
- Don't forget referred pain. Hip pathology can cause pain in the knee.

▨ Marked restriction of movement and/or dramatic bony tenderness suggests a significant problem – especially fracture, septic arthritis and osteomyelitis.

▨ Fever with a limp requires an urgent specialist opinion. Admit to exclude osteomyelitis or septic arthritis.

▨ Beware the fat pubertal boy with groin pain and a limp: slipped femoral epiphysis is likely.

▨ Do not confine your assessment to the hip: for example, abdominal pain, especially appendicitis, can make a child limp.

NOTES:

NUMBNESS AND PARAESTHESIAE

The GP overview

Paraesthesiae and numbness are taken here to mean sensations of tingling, pins-and-needles, subjective numbness, and feelings of cold and heat. They may appear spontaneously or be a result of touching the area of skin concerned. Patients are often alarmed and may make an immediate association with serious disease. The differential is huge but most cases in primary care involve anxiety, nerve entrapment or cerebrovascular disease.

Differential diagnosis

COMMON
- anxiety with hyperventilation
- carpal tunnel (CT) syndrome
- sciatica
- diabetic neuropathy
- cervical spondylosis

OCCASIONAL
- multiple sclerosis and dorsal myelitis
- peripheral polyneuropathy (especially alcohol; also vitamin B_{12} and folate deficiency, iatrogenic, metabolic, connective tissue disorder, malignancy and rare causes such as Guillain–Barré, leprosy)
- stroke and TIA
- trauma/compression involving a peripheral nerve or spinal cord
- migraine with focal neurological signs

RARE
- intramedullary spinal cord tumour
- syringomyelia
- trauma, brain tumour and epilepsy affecting sensory cortex
- hysteria
- vascular: ischaemic heart disease, peripheral vascular disease

Ready reckoner

	Anxiety	CT syndrome	Sciatica	Diabetes	Cervical spondylosis
Associated dizziness	Yes	No	No	No	Possible
Episodic	Yes	Possible	No	Possible	Possible
Associated pain	No	Yes	Yes	Possible	Yes
Worse at night	No	Yes	No	No	Possible
Associated weakness	No	Yes	Yes	No	Possible

Possible investigations

LIKELY: urinalysis, blood sugar or HbA1c.

POSSIBLE: FBC, LFT, γGT, U&E, serum calcium, B$_{12}$ and folate, TFT, nerve conduction studies.

SMALL PRINT: autoimmune screen, cervical spine X-ray, secondary care investigations (MRI/CT scan, lumbar puncture, carotid imaging, angiography, myelography).

- Urinalysis: to pick up glycosuria in undiagnosed diabetes.
- Blood sugar or HbA1c: to confirm diabetes.
- FBC: to look for macrocytosis (sign of alcohol excess or B$_{12}$/folate deficiency). May be anaemia of chronic illness or malignancy.
- LFT and γGT if alcoholic neuropathy suspected.
- Metabolic screen (including U&E, calcium, LFT, B$_{12}$ and folate).
- TFT: hypothyroidism can cause a polyneuropathy or precipitate carpal tunnel syndrome.
- Autoimmune screen: to help diagnose a connective tissue disorder.
- Nerve conduction studies: to confirm a diagnosis of nerve compression prior to surgical treatment.
- X-ray cervical spine: confirms clinical diagnosis of cervical spondylosis, but not really helpful as positive findings common and don't correlate well with symptoms, and the investigation is unlikely to alter the management.
- Secondary care investigations might include: lumbar puncture (MS, Guillain–Barré syndrome), carotid imaging (TIA), CT or MRI scan (spinal pathology or compression, MS, cerebral tumour, syringomyelia), angiography (vascular causes), myelography (cord compression).

TOP TIPS

- Intermittent perioral paraesthesiae are pathognomic of hyperventilation.
- Use a logical approach: a careful history will often reveal the likely underlying problem. For example: well-demarcated area in anatomically explicable distribution – peripheral nerve entrapment; larger area, one limb – root compression; whole side of body – cerebral lesion; hands and feet – peripheral neuropathy; legs alone – cord lesion.

- Wasting of the thenar eminence suggests significant CT syndrome which will require decompression.
- Remember to tell women taking the combined oral contraceptive who develop migraine with focal symptoms to use an alternative method of contraception.

- Sudden and progressive bilateral leg symptoms with sphincter disturbance suggest cord compression: admit immediately.
- Intermittent paraesthesiae in varying distributions – especially with other features, such as vertigo or optic neuritis – suggest MS.
- Patients with TIAs with an 'ABCD2' score of 4 or more should be seen by a specialist within 24 hours; those with lower scores should be seen within 1 week.
- The borders of sensory loss in hysteria are often sharply demarcated and do not correspond to an anatomical pattern.
- Constant, progressive paraesthesiae, especially with other neurological symptoms or signs, suggest significant pathology. Refer urgently.

NOTES:

PROLONGED FEVER

The GP overview

GPs deal with fevers on a daily basis – the vast majority are caused by viruses and are self-limiting. This section deals with a different and much less common scenario: a temperature above normal for 3 weeks or more. It may be continuous or swinging. Many more causes exist than can be named here, but those likeliest in general practice are listed.

Differential diagnosis

COMMON
- glandular fever (GF)
- abscess (anywhere)
- chronic pyelonephritis (recurrent UTI)
- carcinoma (especially bronchial)
- rheumatoid arthritis (RA)

OCCASIONAL
- lymphoma and leukaemia
- systemic lupus erythematosus, polyarteritis nodosa, polymyositis
- Crohn's disease and ulcerative colitis
- drug idiosyncrasies

RARE
- malaria and other tropical diseases
- Lyme disease
- tuberculosis, syphilis
- actinomycosis
- HIV infection: AIDS
- infective endocarditis
- factitious

Ready reckoner

	GF	Abscess	UTI	Carcinoma	RA
Generalised lymphadenopathy	Possible	No	No	Possible	Possible
Local lymphadenopathy	Possible	Yes	No	Possible	No
Frequency of micturition	No	No	Yes	No	No
Rapid weight loss	Possible	Possible	No	Yes	Possible
Joint swelling	No	No	No	Possible	Yes

Possible investigations

LIKELY: FBC, ESR/CRP, LFT, U&E, urinalysis, MSU.

POSSIBLE: Paul–Bunnell test, CXR, autoimmune screen.

SMALL PRINT: faecal calprotectin, blood cultures, malaria films, syphilis serology, HIV test and a variety of other secondary care-based tests.

- FBC, ESR/CRP, U&E, LFT: anaemia will be revealed in a variety of disorders (e.g. malignancy, connective tissue disorders); WCC raised in many inflammatory or infective processes and also some blood dyscrasias. Elevated ESR/CRP a non-specific finding in many of the illnesses listed. Abnormal U&E or LFT may point to an underlying renal or hepatic problem.
- Urinalysis, MSU: may be proteinuria, haematuria and evidence of infection in chronic pyelonephritis.
- Paul–Bunnell test: may be positive in glandular fever.
- CXR: will show signs of malignancy (e.g. lung, lymphoma), occult infection and TB.
- Autoimmune screen: may suggest a connective tissue disorder.
- Faecal calprotectin: if symptoms suggest possible IBD.
- Secondary care-based tests: a number of tests may be performed after referral to the specialist in cases which remain obscure after initial assessment and investigation. These include further microbiological tests (e.g. stool, blood cultures), blood tests (e.g. for malaria, syphilis and HIV), isotope scans, ultrasound and CT scans (for occult infection or malignancy), tuberculin testing (for possible TB) and esoteric tests for tropical diseases.

TOP TIPS

- Prolonged fever is usually an uncommon presentation of a common disorder (unless there has been recent travel), so review the situation regularly and encourage the patient to report new symptoms, which may help reveal the diagnosis.
- Refer early if the patient is unwell or has lost weight; if not, arrange initial investigations yourself.
- Don't always accept self-reporting of this symptom at face value. Flushing or sweating may be misreported as 'fever'. If in doubt, get the patient to record the temperature over a period of time.

- Always take a travel history, and specifically enquire about insect bites and compliance with antimalarial therapy. Remember, too, occupation and recent contact with infectious illness.

Red flags

- Tuberculosis is rare but on the increase in the UK. Consider this diagnosis, particularly in Asian immigrants and vagrants.
- Itching with prolonged pyrexia suggests leukaemia or lymphoma.
- Refer to a tropical medicine centre a patient with PUO who has recently been abroad somewhere exotic – in such a case, the differential is much wider and the possibility of an obscure pathology therefore much greater.
- Factitious prolonged fever is rare, but possibly more common among health staff; beware the health worker with apparent fever but who never feels hot and who never appears unwell, especially if basic investigations are all normal.
- Don't forget the possibility of infective endocarditis in a patient with a cardiac murmur.

NOTES:

SWOLLEN GLANDS

The GP overview

There are very many causes of swollen glands (lymphadenopathy), but in general it is possible to narrow the list of possible causes down to a manageable few by careful history and examination. Age, geography (or travel history) and distribution of enlarged glands have a considerable influence on the differential diagnosis.

Differential diagnosis

COMMON
- local infection (e.g. URTI, tonsillitis)
- generalised viral infection (e.g. glandular fever, rubella)
- malignancy: secondary metastasis
- white cell malignancy: lymphoma, leukaemia, myeloma
- septicaemia

OCCASIONAL
- sarcoid
- cat scratch fever (especially in children)
- rubella/measles
- SLE
- rheumatoid arthritis
- tropical/subtropical sexually transmitted infection: lymphogranuloma venereum (LGV), granuloma inguinale (GI)

RARE
- syphilis (primary or secondary)
- HIV: AIDS and AIDS-related complex (ARC)
- tuberculosis
- tropical infections: leprosy, filariasis, trypanosomiasis, tularaemia
- drug reactions (e.g. phenytoin, penicillins, sulphonamides)

Ready reckoner

	Local infection	General viral	Metastases	WC malignancy	Septicaemia
Tender nodes	Yes	Yes	No	Possible	Possible
Persistent (>6 weeks)	No	No	Yes	Yes	No
Regional nodes only	Yes	No	Yes	Possible	No
Firm splenomegaly	No	Possible	No	Possible	No
Night sweats	No	Possible	Possible	Yes	Possible

Possible investigations

LIKELY: none if localised; FBC and ESR/CRP if generalised.

POSSIBLE: Paul–Bunnell test, CXR, acute and convalescent sera, HIV testing, lymph node biopsy.

SMALL PRINT: autoimmune blood tests, syphilis serology, cultures and scrapings for LGV and GI, Kveim test, CT scan, indirect fluorescent antibody blood test for *Bartonella henselae*.

- ☑ FBC: atypical lymphocytes reflect acute viral infection; many of the causes listed will result in a raised WCC and ESR/CRP. Hb may be low in malignancy and connective tissue disease; WCC and film may show evidence of lymphoma or leukaemia.
- ☑ Paul–Bunnell test: to confirm glandular fever.
- ☑ CXR: may reveal carcinoma, TB, lymphoma, sarcoid and the source of septicaemia.
- ☑ Serology: acute and convalescent sera may confirm specific viral infection.
- ☑ Kveim test for sarcoid.
- ☑ Abdominal and chest CT scan is a sensitive test to detect pelvic, para-aortic, mesenteric, hilar or paratracheal node enlargement (e.g. in lymphoma).
- ☑ Autoimmune blood tests: may help in diagnosis of connective tissue disorder.
- ☑ Culture/scrapings (GUM clinic): for LGV and GI.
- ☑ Syphilis serology, HIV testing: for syphilis and AIDS.
- ☑ Indirect fluorescent antibody test for *B. henselae*: this is the causative organism in cat scratch disease.
- ☑ Lymph node biopsy may be necessary to reach a definitive diagnosis.

TOP TIPS

- ☑ Normal cervical lymph nodes are often palpable in children; they swell with URTIs and may be presented by anxious parents fearing significant disease.
- ☑ Remember geography: a young adult from the UK with persistent cervical nodes is likely to have Epstein–Barr virus (EBV) infection while, in Africa, the likeliest diagnosis would be tuberculosis. Swollen groin glands in the latter group might be caused by LGV or GI.
- ☑ Patients often attach great significance to swollen glands. It is worth explaining that lymphadenopathy usually represents a normal part of the immune system's defence against infection and does not in itself require attention from the doctor unless there are unusual features.

☑ Unexplained and persistent cervical lymphadenopathy in the middle-aged and elderly should prompt urgent ENT assessment to exclude nasopharyngeal carcinoma.

☑ An enlarged left supraclavicular node (Troisier's) in a patient with weight loss suggests gastrointestinal carcinoma.

☑ Generalised, persistent lymph nodes with weight loss and sweats in a young adult suggest glandular fever, lymphoma or AIDS.

☑ A slowly enlarging, non-tender cervical node in an unusual site is likely to be malignant.

NOTES:

THIRST OR DRY MOUTH

The GP overview

The complaint of thirst rings alarm bells in doctor and patient alike. Diabetes clearly needs to be excluded but the differential may need to be extended beyond this in the light of negative initial tests. Dry mouth tends to create less concern but can sometimes herald significant pathology and may be a serious nuisance to the patient.

Differential diagnosis

COMMON
- diabetes mellitus
- dehydration
- medication (e.g. tricyclic antidepressants, antihistamines)
- mouth breathing (usually through nasal blockage)
- anxiety

OCCASIONAL
- normality (children sometimes presented because 'they are always thirsty')
- smoking
- excess alcohol
- Sjögren's syndrome
- hypercalcaemia
- chronic kidney disease (CKD)

RARE
- pregnancy (common condition but rarely causes significant thirst)
- compulsive water drinking
- sickle-cell disease
- previous head/neck irradiation

Ready reckoner

	Diabetes mellitus	Dehydration	Medication	Mouth breathing	Anxiety
Polyuria/frequency	Yes	No	No	No	Possible
Generally unwell	Possible	Yes	Possible	No	Possible
Difficulty breathing through nose	No	No	No	Yes	No
Symptom intermittent	No	No	Possible	Possible	Possible
Clinically dehydrated	Possible	Yes	No	No	No

Possible investigations

LIKELY: urinalysis, fasting blood glucose or HbA1c.

POSSIBLE: FBC, ESR/CRP, U&E, calcium, rheumatoid factor and other autoantibody screen.

SMALL PRINT: serum and urine osmolality, sickle-cell screen.

- ◪ Urinalysis: glycosuria in diabetes, specific gravity raised in dehydration and reduced in diabetes insipidus and compulsive water drinking, may be proteinuria and/or microscopic haematuria in CKD.
- ◪ Fasting blood glucose or HbA1c: to definitively diagnose diabetes.
- ◪ FBC/ESR: Hb may be reduced and ESR elevated in Sjögren's linked to connective tissue disorder; Hb may also be reduced in CKD.
- ◪ U&E: may suggest dehydration or CKD.
- ◪ Calcium: elevated in hypercalcaemia.
- ◪ Rheumatoid factor and other autoantibodies: Sjögren's may be linked to rheumatoid arthritis, SLE or other connective tissue disease.
- ◪ Serum and urine osmolality: serum osmolality raised and urine osmolality low in diabetes insipidus; in compulsive water drinking, serum osmolality low.
- ◪ Sickle-cell screen: to detect sickle-cell anaemia.

TOP TIPS

- ◪ The assessment of thirst does not stop at the exclusion of diabetes mellitus – consider other causes.
- ◪ Intermittent dry mouth in an anxious individual also reporting episodic perioral paraesthesiae is likely to be caused by anxiety – perhaps aggravated by certain medications the patient might be taking for the problem.
- ◪ Do not underestimate the complaint of dry mouth, especially in the elderly – it can cause significant distress.
- ◪ Remember hypercalcaemia, particularly in palliative care patients – this is a potentially remediable cause of troublesome thirst.

◪ Children who are 'always thirsty', have been like that for as long as the parents can remember and are otherwise well will not have diabetes – though the parents may feel short-changed if this isn't tested for.

Red flags

◪ In the acute presentation of thirst, it is essential to exclude diabetes immediately – a very high glucose level with ketonuria will require admission.

◪ Beware the thirsty elderly patient with an acute illness, particularly if the patient is on ACE inhibitors – he or she may be significantly dehydrated and developing renal failure.

◪ Dry eyes and joint swellings in association with a dry mouth may indicate Sjögren's.

◪ Beware that the elderly with diabetes may complain of dry mouth rather than thirst.

NOTES:

TIREDNESS

The GP overview

Feeling tired all the time is such a common presenting symptom that 'TATT' has become the universal GP acronym. In around 85% of first consultations the cause is apparent by the end. Although the vast majority turn out to have a non-organic cause, it is clearly important not to get lulled into ignoring important physical illness. A structured approach can turn this heartsink calling card into a rewarding and successful consultation.

Differential diagnosis

COMMON
- ☑ true depressive illness
- ☑ stress (overwork, young children, boredom, etc.)
- ☑ anaemia
- ☑ acute post-viral fatigue
- ☑ hypothyroidism

OCCASIONAL
- ☑ diabetes mellitus
- ☑ iron deficiency (in the absence of anaemia)
- ☑ coeliac disease
- ☑ any cause of insomnia (see p. 80)
- ☑ chronic post-viral fatigue syndrome ('ME')
- ☑ major organ failure (heart, liver, kidney)
- ☑ hyperthyroidism
- ☑ substance misuse
- ☑ drug therapy (β-blockers, diuretics)

RARE
- ☑ malignant disease
- ☑ chronic infection (e.g. TB, hepatitis, HIV)
- ☑ chronic neurological disorders (Parkinson's disease, myasthenia gravis, MS, motor neurone disease)
- ☑ other endocrine disorders and deficiency states (e.g. Addison's disease, hypo- or hypercalcaemia, hyponatraemia, hypokalaemia)
- ☑ connective tissue diseases (RA, polymyalgia rheumatica (PMR), SLE)
- ☑ carbon monoxide poisoning

224

Ready reckoner

	Depression	Stress	Anaemia	Post-viral	Hypothyroidism
Diurnal variation	Yes	Possible	No	No	No
Identifiable life event triggers	Possible	Yes	No	No	No
Recent illness	Possible	Possible	Possible	Yes	No
Mucosal/nailbed pallor	No	No	Yes	No	Possible
Cold, dry skin	No	No	Possible	No	Yes

Possible investigations

LIKELY: urinalysis, FBC, blood glucose or HbA1c, TFT.

POSSIBLE: ESR/CRP, U&E, LFT, ferritin, calcium, anti-endomysial and anti-gliadin antibodies.

SMALL PRINT: CXR, autoantibody screen, further blood tests as indicated such as HIV, glandular fever test, hepatitis serology.

- Urinalysis: simple screen for diabetes and renal disease.
- Blood glucose or HbA1c: for diabetes.
- TFT for hypo- or hyperthyroidism.
- FBC: the anaemias, infection and alcohol abuse.
- ESR/CRP: raised in a host of causes; not diagnostic but suggests a possible underlying physical cause.
- U&E: deranged in renal failure, hyponatraemia, hypokalaemia and Addison's disease.
- LFT: for liver disease (malignancy, alcohol abuse and hepatitis).
- Ferritin: iron deficiency may cause tiredness in the absence of anaemia.
- Calcium: hyper- or hypocalcaemia may cause tiredness.
- Anti-endomysial and anti-gliadin antibodies: will suggest a diagnosis of coeliac disease.
- Autoantibody screen: for connective tissue disease.
- Further blood tests: these will be dictated by the clinical picture and might include HIV, glandular fever or hepatitis testing.
- CXR: may reveal malignancy, cardiac failure or TB.

TOP TIPS

- Tiredness as a presenting symptom, in the absence of other significant volunteered symptoms – particularly weight loss or gain – is unlikely to have a physical cause.
- The longer tiredness has been a problem, the less likely you will find *any* remediable cause.
- Make eye contact with the patient and shake hands – your first impressions as to whether or not the patient is actually 'ill' are likely to prove correct, and may give early clues to easily overlooked causes such as Parkinson's disease.
- If you suspect depression, enquire directly about relevant symptoms – you do not have to 'exclude' physical illness before making a presumptive diagnosis of this sort.

- Investigations ordered are often more therapeutic than diagnostic.
- Ask about other household members' health and well-being. Carbon monoxide poisoning would be likely to affect them too.
- Do not be too trigger-happy with the usual 'blood screen'. Many patients 'promised' blood tests if their symptoms persist another month do not return.

- Take tiredness associated with weight loss seriously – this combination suggests malignant disease or hyperthyroidism.
- Don't miss depressive illness by being coy in enquiry or colluding with patient denial.
- Don't miss easy-to-find signs when physical illness seems a real possibility – check pulse rate, mucous membranes for pallor, lymph nodes, chest and abdomen.
- Consider a rare cause if the symptoms progress and the patient starts to look unwell.

NOTES:

TREMOR

The GP overview

This is rhythmic movement of parts of the body. There are three clinical types: rest tremor (worst at rest), postural tremor (worst in a fixed posture, e.g. outstretched arms) and intention tremor (worst during voluntary movement). Tremor may be noticed by the GP during an assessment for some other problem, or it may be the presenting symptom. In the latter case, the patient may be embarrassed by the lack of 'self-control', so a sympathetic approach is important.

Differential diagnosis

COMMON
- anxiety
- thyrotoxicosis
- drug withdrawal (e.g. opiates, benzodiazepines, alcohol)
- benign essential tremor (familial)
- Parkinson's disease

OCCASIONAL
- adverse drug reaction (e.g. phenothiazines, β-agonists)
- carbon dioxide retention (e.g. COPD)
- multiple sclerosis (MS)
- cerebellar ataxia: many causes, including tumour, acoustic neuroma, Friedreich's ataxia, CVA, abscess

RARE
- fulminant hepatic failure
- Wilson's disease
- tertiary syphilis
- hysterical: usually restricted to one limb and is very gross
- meningoencephalitis

Ready reckoner

	Anxiety	Thyrotoxicosis	Drug withdrawal	Benign essential	Parkinson's disease
Rest tremor	No	No	No	No	Yes
Suppressed by alcohol	Possible	No	Possible	Yes	No
Otherwise well	Possible	No	No	Yes	No
Tachycardia	Yes	Yes	Possible	No	No
Bradykinesia	No	No	No	No	Yes

Possible investigations

LIKELY: TFT.

POSSIBLE: FBC, LFT.

SMALL PRINT: syphilis serology and, in secondary care, MRI scan, lumbar puncture, visual evoked response, serum caeruloplasmin/blood copper, blood gases.

- ◪ FBC: macrocytosis in chronic alcohol excess.
- ◪ LFT: for evidence of alcohol abuse or liver failure.
- ◪ TFT: if hyperthyroidism suspected.
- ◪ MRI most sensitive test for picking up CNS demyelination and tumours (e.g. cerebellar).
- ◪ Lumbar puncture: CSF electrophoresis may show oligoclonal bands in MS, or evidence of meningoencephalitis.
- ◪ Visual evoked response: prolonged in MS.
- ◪ Syphilis serology: in suspected syphilis.
- ◪ Blood gases: will reveal carbon dioxide retention.
- ◪ Serum caeruloplasmin/blood copper: to diagnose Wilson's disease.

TOP TIPS

- ◪ Patients who present with their tremor are invariably worried about significant disease, especially Parkinson's disease. Ensure that these anxieties are resolved during the consultation.
- ◪ Essential tremor is characteristically suppressed by a small dose of alcohol. This can be a useful pointer from the history.
- ◪ A tremor can have more than one cause and may not necessarily follow the neat patterns described, especially in the elderly.
- ◪ The tremor of early Parkinson's disease usually causes the patient few problems. It may therefore be noticed by the doctor when the patient presents with other symptoms, or be presented by concerned relatives or friends.

- Have a low threshold for arranging TFT: anxiety can closely mimic thyrotoxicosis and vice versa.
- Parkinson's disease may well present with a consultation for frequent falls. Look for other signs such as mask face, small handwriting, slow movement, festinant gait and difficulty rising from chair.
- Think of alcohol problems in isolated middle-aged and elderly men developing postural tremor.
- Intention tremor with nystagmus or dysarthria suggests significant cerebellar pathology.

NOTES:

WEIGHT GAIN

The GP overview

By far the commonest cause of this problem is simple obesity. This is 50% commoner in women, who also present more often than men. It may be the primary problem presented or it may be a 'while I'm here' symptom – either way, it tends to be viewed as a 'heartsink' symptom, as such patients may have unrealistic expectations of what the doctor can achieve.

Differential diagnosis

COMMON
- simple obesity (usually hereditary component with poor diet and lack of exercise)
- hypothyroidism
- pregnancy
- oedema of any cause (e.g. cardiac failure, renal failure, hepatic failure)
- alcohol excess

OCCASIONAL
- menopause
- iatrogenic (e.g. steroids, insulin, sulphonylureas, oestrogen, pizotifen)
- polycystic ovary syndrome
- large single ovarian cyst
- physical or mental disability restricting activity (e.g. CVA, Down's syndrome)

RARE
- anabolic steroid abuse
- Cushing's syndrome
- hypothalamic lesion or hypopituitarism
- insulinoma
- rare genetic syndromes such as Prader–Willi syndrome

Ready reckoner

	Simple obesity	Hypothyroidism	Pregnancy	Oedema	Alcohol
Pitting oedema	Possible	No	Possible	Yes	Possible
Only abdominal girth increased	No	No	Yes	No	Possible
Long history	Yes	Possible	No	Possible	Possible
Palpable liver	No	No	No	Possible	Possible
Otherwise well	Yes	Possible	Possible	No	No

Possible investigations

LIKELY: TFT.

POSSIBLE: urinalysis, FBC, LFT, U&E, pregnancy test, cardiac investigations if the cause is possible cardiac failure, pelvic ultrasound.

SMALL PRINT: secondary care investigations for endocrine dysfunction.

- Urinalysis: proteinuria may be present in oedema caused by underlying renal disease.
- FBC: anaemia may precipitate cardiac failure; MCV raised in hypothyroidism and alcohol excess.
- TFT: will reveal hypothyroidism.
- U&E: deranged in renal failure and Cushing's syndrome.
- LFT: to check for liver failure, evidence of alcohol abuse and hypoproteinaemic states.
- Pregnancy test: to exclude pregnancy if this is a possibility.
- Pelvic ultrasound: will confirm ascites, ovarian cysts and pregnancy.
- Cardiac investigations: CXR, ECG, BNP and echocardiography if the underlying cause is possible cardiac failure.
- Secondary care investigations for endocrine dysfunction: for insulinoma, hypopituitarism, Cushing's syndrome.

TOP TIPS

- Patients presenting with weight gain, especially if it is a long-term or fluctuating problem, usually have a clear agenda of their own – such as wanting a blood test or drug treatment. Much time can be wasted giving unwanted advice about diet and exercise which the patient will have heard before. Establish the patient's agenda early in the consultation.
- Parents anxious about weight gain in their children often want to be reassured that the child's 'glands' are normal. If the child's height is in proportion to its weight, or the parents have a similar physiognomy, and the child is otherwise well, it is highly unlikely that there is an underlying cause.
- Patients with Down's syndrome have a relatively high prevalence of hypothyroidism –

consider this possibility if a patient with Down's syndrome experiences inexplicable weight gain.

☑ Investigation is usually clinically unnecessary, but may be useful to clear the way to dealing with the real cause.

Red flags

☑ Correction of hypothyroidism may not solve a weight gain problem, merely unmask an underlying simple obesity. Don't falsely raise expectations.

☑ Establish whether the weight gain is diffuse or whether there is predominantly abdominal swelling. The latter may indicate pregnancy, ascites or a large ovarian cyst.

☑ Recent onset of weight gain in an elderly patient suggests probable congestive cardiac failure or possible hypothyroidism.

☑ Young women may not consider, or accept, a diagnosis of pregnancy as a cause of their weight gain. Arrange a pregnancy test if in any doubt.

☑ The yield from routine blood tests is low – but consider investigation if the patient is unwell or the history atypical.

NOTES:

WEIGHT LOSS

The GP overview

The significance of weight loss should not be underestimated: in about one-third of patients, there is no specific cause, but in the rest, a serious underlying pathology is found. The minority of these are psychiatric; 90% have organic illness. Thorough assessment from the start is the rule.

Differential diagnosis

COMMON
- 'normal' stressful life events without psychiatric illness (e.g. changing job, divorce, redundancy, bereavement, exam pressure)
- clinical depressive illness
- eating disorders: anorexia nervosa and bulimia nervosa
- hyperthyroidism: thyrotoxicosis and iatrogenic (excess thyroid replacement)
- malignancy anywhere

OCCASIONAL
- anxiety (of whatever cause)
- any terminal illness (e.g. malignancy, motor neurone disease)
- substance misuse: alcohol, opiates, amphetamines, laxatives
- organ failure: cardiac, renal and hepatic
- undiagnosed diabetes mellitus
- chronic inflammatory conditions (e.g. RA, SLE)
- gastrointestinal disease (e.g. peptic ulcer, inflammatory bowel disease, coeliac disease, parasites)

RARE
- any chronic infection (especially tuberculosis)
- endocrine: Addison's disease, phaeochromocytoma
- AIDS
- malnutrition (rare in developed countries, common worldwide)

Ready reckoner

	Normal stress	Depression	Eating disorders	Hyperthyroidism	Malignancy
Mild anxiety	Yes	Possible	No	No	No
Loss of appetite	Possible	Yes	No	No	Yes
Distorted body image	No	No	Yes	No	No
Recurrent problem	Yes	Possible	Possible	Possible	No
Severe malaise	No	Yes	No	Possible	Yes

Possible investigations

LIKELY: urinalysis, FBC, ESR/CRP, TFT, U&E, LFT, CXR, blood glucose or HbA1c.

POSSIBLE: autoimmune screen, HIV test, bowel investigations such as faecal calprotectin or anti-endomysial and anti-gliadin antibodies, other hospital-based investigations.

SMALL PRINT: none.

- Urinalysis: for possible undiagnosed diabetes; proteinuria in renal failure.
- FBC and ESR/CRP: Hb may be reduced and ESR/CRP elevated in malignancy and any chronic disorder.
- U&E: abnormal in renal failure and sometimes in eating disorders; sodium reduced, potassium and urea elevated in Addison's disease.
- TFT: will confirm hyperthyroidism.
- LFT: deranged in alcoholism and liver disease.
- Blood glucose or HbA1c: to confirm diabetes.
- Autoimmune screen: may be helpful in suspected connective tissue disorder.
- HIV test: if AIDS suspected.
- Bowel investigations such as faecal calprotectin or anti-endomysial and anti-gliadin antibodies: if IBD or coeliac disease suspected.
- CXR: may reveal carcinoma, TB, lymphadenopathy or cardiac failure.
- Other investigations (usually hospital-based) may be required according to the symptoms accompanying the weight loss and the results of preliminary investigations.

TOP TIPS

- Weight loss needs to be taken seriously but can be complex and time-consuming to assess. If presented as a 'by the way' at the end of a consultation for some other matter, it is reasonable to reverse the normal approach by arranging basic blood tests and urinalysis first, and booking a follow-up appointment, with the results, for a more complete assessment.
- Establish whether episodes of weight loss have happened before. Patients, or their records, may indicate, for example, that they always lose weight when stressed.
- Check that the patient really has lost weight. The history may not be clear, and there is

often a record available (e.g. new patient check or health promotion data) of previous weight.

☑ Look at the patient. The obviously cachectic will have significant disease and require urgent and thorough investigation.

☑ Rapid weight loss with malaise and respiratory or gastrointestinal symptoms strongly suggest a physical cause.

☑ Think of eating disorders in young females: look for acid dental erosion on palatal surfaces of upper teeth as a giveaway sign of recurrent vomiting.

☑ Weight loss in a child is caused either by significant organic pathology or emotional abuse. Look out for signs of non-accidental injury (NAI) during physical examination.

☑ Depression with weight loss is a difficult problem; it may be the primary cause or the change in mood may be secondary to some physical illness. Either way, don't overlook significant depression while you arrange investigations; there is nothing to be lost in starting antidepressants while you continue to exclude a physical cause, so long as you explain your strategy to the patient.

NOTES:

GENITAL

Erectile dysfunction

Haemospermia

Painful intercourse

Penile pain

Penile ulceration/sores

Scrotal swelling

Testicular pain

Vaginal discharge

Vulval irritation

Vulval swelling

Vulval ulceration/sores

ERECTILE DYSFUNCTION

The GP overview

This is the partial or complete failure to achieve a satisfactory erection. The inability to ejaculate (ejaculatory erectile dysfunction) is not dealt with here. It presents fairly often to GPs and will probably do so increasingly frequently as new treatments are developed and publicised.

Differential diagnosis

COMMON
- depression/anxiety
- excessive alcohol intake
- relationship dysfunction
- vascular: arterial insufficiency (arteriopathy) or excessive venous drainage
- iatrogenic (e.g. prostatic cancer treatments, hypotensives, some antidepressants)

OCCASIONAL
- testosterone deficiency (may be primary or secondary)
- diabetic autonomic neuropathy
- trauma: pelvic or spinal fracture, trauma to penis, post-TURP
- anatomical: phimosis, tight frenulum
- excessive cigarette smoking
- Peyronie's disease
- drug abuse (e.g. heroin, amphetamines)

RARE
- fetishism (erection only possible with unusual stimuli)
- spinal cord compression: tumour
- thrombosis of a corpus cavernosum
- neurological: tabes dorsalis, multiple sclerosis

Ready reckoner

	Depression/anxiety	Alcohol	Relationship dysfunction	Vascular	Drugs
TATT/sleep problem	Yes	Possible	Possible	No	No
Occasional only	Possible	No	Yes	No	No
Full morning erection	Yes	No	Yes	No	No
Reduced foot pulses	No	No	No	Yes	No
Taking medication	Possible	No	No	No	Yes

Possible investigations

LIKELY: urinalysis.

POSSIBLE: blood sugar or HbA1c, FBC, LFT, endocrine assays (testosterone, prolactin, FSH/LH, TSH), cholesterol.

SMALL PRINT: Doppler flow studies, angiography, intracorporeal prostaglandin injection test, MRI scanning – all likely to be specialist initiated.

- Urinalysis: an essential easy screen for undiagnosed diabetes.
- Blood sugar or HbA1c: to confirm diabetes.
- FBC and LFT possibly helpful in alcohol excess (raised MCV and possible LFT abnormalities).
- Testosterone levels reduced in primary or secondary hypogonadism. Prolactin, FSH/LH and TSH check pituitary function. Erectile dysfunction may be a sign of cardiovascular disease – so in certain patients a cholesterol level would be warranted.
- Doppler flow studies of superficial and deep penile arterial flow assess arterial sufficiency. Angiography may be necessary if symptoms suggest significant lower limb arterial insufficiency associated with impotence.
- Intracorporeal prostaglandin injection test: immediate and prolonged response indicates neurological problems. Good initial response with rapid failure indicates excessive venous drainage.
- Possible neurological causes will occasionally require further investigation (e.g. MRI scanning for cord lesions or MS).

TOP TIPS

- Establish whether the patient can get an erection at any time (e.g. early morning). If he can, then the cause is unlikely to be organic. Take a positive approach – many psychological causes are transient.
- Don't be too quick to diagnose anxiety as the underlying problem. This may be the effect, rather than the cause, of the impotence.
- Erectile dysfunction is often presented as a 'by the way' or 'while I'm here' symptom.

The temptation is to invite the patient to book a further appointment, but bear in mind that this may represent a lost opportunity to help, as he may not return.

◪ Demonstrate that you are taking the problem seriously – for example, by performing an appropriate examination or by inviting the patient's partner to attend a subsequent appointment.

Red flags

◪ Sudden onset of erectile dysfunction with saddle anaesthesia and sphincter disturbance indicates a cauda equina lesion. Refer urgently.

◪ An erection which is consistently lost after a predictable period is likely to be organic – probably vascular – in origin.

◪ Early morning headache and visual disturbance suggests a pituitary fossa tumour.

◪ Do not forget that alcohol and drug abuse are possible causes. Look in the notes for clues and make specific enquiry, as these problems are unlikely to be volunteered.

◪ Erectile dysfunction may well be a marker for vascular disease elsewhere. Extend your assessment as appropriate.

NOTES:

HAEMOSPERMIA

The GP overview

This is an uncommon presentation – but one we may see increasingly frequently as men become less reticent about coming to the doctor. As with any symptom involving leakage of blood, anxiety levels tend to run high. This shouldn't transfer to the GP, though – it is unusual for the symptom to have a sinister cause.

Differential diagnosis

COMMON
- unknown (at least 50%; the majority are probably secondary to forgotten or unnoticed trauma)
- prostatitis
- post-operative (prostate surgery, biopsy or extracorporeal shock wave lithotripsy)
- genito-urinary infection (epididymo-orchitis, urethritis, UTI)
- trauma (to testicles or perineum)

OCCASIONAL
- blood clotting disorder or anticoagulation
- calculi in the prostate
- carcinoma: prostate, testicles, bladder or seminal vesicles

RARE
- tuberculosis
- schistosomiasis
- malignant hypertension
- structural problems (such as urethral strictures or polyps)

Ready reckoner

	Unknown	Prostatitis	Post-op	GU infection	Trauma
Persistent	Possible	Possible	No	Possible	No
Recent surgical intervention	No	Possible	Yes	Possible	No
Recent trauma	Possible	No	No	No	Yes
Urinary tract symptoms	No	Possible	Possible	Yes	No
Prostate markedly tender on PR	No	Yes	Possible	No	No

Possible investigations

LIKELY: urinalysis, MSU.

POSSIBLE: FBC, ESR/CRP, PSA, urethral swab.

SMALL PRINT: INR, clotting screen, seminal fluid culture, transrectal ultrasound, prostate biopsy, urethroscopy.

- Urinalysis: protein, nitrites, leucocytes and possible haematuria in any genito-urinary infection or prostatitis. Haematuria possible in malignancy and schistosomiasis.
- MSU: to confirm infection and identify pathogen.
- FBC and ESR/CRP: WCC may be elevated in infection; Hb may be reduced and ESR/CRP raised in malignancy; ESR/CRP also raised in infection.
- PSA: the pros and cons of this test might be discussed as a pointer to prostatic carcinoma.
- Urethral swab: if urethritis suspected (best taken at GUM clinic).
- INR, clotting screen: if patient on warfarin or a bleeding disorder suspected.
- Other investigations (usually hospital-based): these might include seminal fluid culture to investigate deep-seated infection; transrectal ultrasound and prostatic biopsy for detailed investigation of prostate; urethroscopy/cystoscopy if felt to be a structural urethral or bladder problem.

TOP TIPS

- A frank and open approach, using plain language, is important for the patient to feel comfortable and capable of describing an accurate history.
- Do not underestimate the patient's level of anxiety – and ensure it's properly addressed. Most men with this symptom are convinced they have serious pathology.
- The approach with this symptom has more to do with deciding on further action than establishing a precise diagnosis. This is because assessment in primary care rarely reveals any underlying pathology – management is more likely to be influenced by the patient's age and the history than the clinical findings (see below).
- Men under the age of 40 with short-lived symptoms do not require referral, as the chance of significant pathology is miniscule. Older men – and those with persistent or recurrent

haemospermia, or abnormalities on initial assessment – require referral for further assessment.

- A serious underlying cause is rare but should be considered in men over the age of 40 who have more than one episode.
- The chances of significant pathology are increased by the finding of microscopic haematuria – refer these cases.

NOTES:

PAINFUL INTERCOURSE

The GP overview

This term is taken to apply to women. It causes much misery and may be embarrassing for a woman to discuss with her doctor. As a result, it may be the 'hidden agenda', presenting as a non-existent 'discharge' or vague 'soreness down below'. Alternatively, it may be the underlying cause of a presentation of infertility or stress. Tact and sensitivity are the most valuable diagnostic and therapeutic tools in these situations.

Differential diagnosis

COMMON
- pure vaginismus: psychogenic spasm and dryness
- vulvovaginitis (especially infection, e.g. bacterial or fungal vaginosis, ulceration, bartholinitis)
- menopausal vaginal dryness (atrophic vaginitis)
- endometriosis
- pelvic inflammatory disease (PID) and cervicitis

OCCASIONAL
- post-partum perineal repair
- pelvic congestion (pelvic pain syndrome)
- fibroid and retroverted uterus, ovaries in pouch of Douglas
- pelvic adhesions (post-surgical or PID)
- cystitis, urethritis

RARE
- congenital abnormality
- large ovarian cyst or tumour
- vulval dysplasia
- urethral caruncle
- unruptured hymen
- anal fissure, thrombosed piles, perianal abscess

Ready reckoner

	Vaginismus	Vulvovaginitis	Atrophic vaginitis	Endometriosis	PID
Abnormal discharge	No	Yes	Possible	No	Possible
Deep dyspareunia	No	No	No	Yes	Yes
Heavy painful periods	No	No	No	Yes	Possible
Vaginal dryness	Yes	No	Yes	No	No
Tight introitus O/E	Yes	No	No	No	No

Possible investigations

LIKELY: high vaginal/cervical swabs.

POSSIBLE: urinalysis, MSU, urethral swab, ultrasound, laparoscopy (in secondary care).

SMALL PRINT: FBC, ESR/CRP, vulval biopsy (secondary care).

- Urinalysis for nitrite, pus cells and blood useful to rule out UTI.
- MSU will help guide treatment in UTI.
- If abnormal discharge, take high vaginal and cervical swabs to establish nature of pathogen. Urethral swab useful if possible urethritis (usually at genito-urinary medicine (GUM) clinic).
- FBC may show raised WCC in chronic PID.
- ESR/CRP elevated in PID.
- Pelvic ultrasound can define lie of the uterus and ovaries, presence of cysts and gross endometriosis.
- Investigations after referral may include laparoscopy (e.g. for endometriosis and PID) and vulval biopsy (for suspected dysplasia).

TOP TIPS

- Superficial dyspareunia (pain at the introitus) is usually caused by infection, vaginismus or atrophy; deep dyspareunia (deep pain) may be caused by pelvic pathology.
- If a sexually transmitted infection could be the cause, refer to a GUM clinic: these are best equipped for thorough screening, counselling and contact tracing.
- The patient complaining that her 'vagina feels too small' to accommodate her partner's penis probably has vaginismus.
- Deep dyspareunia which is long-standing and positional is 'collision' dyspareunia and is very unlikely to be due to significant pathology.
- Deep dyspareunia usually resolves immediately on withdrawal; if it lasts a day or two after intercourse, it may well have a psychological basis.

Red flags

☑ Relationship problems may cause dislike of intercourse which presents as pain. Disharmony may be the cause rather than result of the problem.

☑ Cyclical dyspareunia with generalised pelvic pain and heavy, painful periods suggest endometriosis or PID: refer for gynaecological opinion.

☑ Pelvic tumour is rare in this context, but consider this possibility in the older woman presenting with deep dyspareunia of recent onset.

☑ Examine the menopausal or perimenopausal woman complaining of persistent superficial dyspareunia – vulval dysplasia, rather than atrophic vaginitis, may be the cause.

NOTES:

PENILE PAIN

The GP overview

Pain in the penis occurs not just as a result of local causes, but also by referral from remote lesions. It frequently generates embarrassment for the patient, who may also be frightened that he has a sexually transmitted disease. The diagnosis will often be clear after a carefully taken history and appropriate examination.

Differential diagnosis

COMMON
- balanitis (fungal, bacterial or allergic)
- acute urethritis
- phimosis (e.g. balanitis xerotica obliterans)
- urinary calculus (at any point in ureter or urethra)
- prostatitis/prostatic abscess

OCCASIONAL
- herpes simplex (and rarely zoster)
- carcinoma of bladder or prostate
- trauma: torn frenulum, zipper injury, urethral injury or foreign body
- acute cystitis
- Peyronie's disease (pain usually on erection)
- paraphimosis
- tight frenulum

RARE
- anal fissure/inflamed haemorrhoid
- carcinoma of penis
- carcinoma of rectum/anus
- tuberculosis of urinary tract
- schistosomiasis (*Schistosoma haematobium*): common in Africa and the Middle East

Ready reckoner

	Balanitis	Prostatitis	Calculus	Phimosis	Urethritis
Dysuria	Possible	Possible	Possible	Possible	Yes
Discharge	Yes	Possible	No	Possible	Yes
Rectal pain	No	Yes	Possible	No	Possible
Haematuria	No	Possible	Yes	No	Possible
Tender glans	Yes	No	No	Possible	No

Possible investigations

LIKELY: urinalysis, MSU, swabs.

POSSIBLE: FBC, ESR/CRP, PSA.

SMALL PRINT: IVU, cystoscopy, terminal stream urine.

- Urinalysis: may reveal proteinuria, haematuria, pus cells and nitrites in the presence of infection; haematuria alone with a stone. Will also reveal glycosuria in the previously undiagnosed diabetic (may present with candidal balanitis).
- MSU (for MC&S): to establish pathogen in UTI (may also reveal infective agent in prostatitis).
- Swabs for microbiology: urethral swab if urethritis likely (best performed at GUM clinic). In balanitis with discharge, a swab may help guide treatment.
- FBC and ESR/CRP: WCC and ESR/CRP raised in significant infection and inflammation (e.g. prostatitis or prostatic abscess). ESR/CRP may be raised in malignancy.
- PSA: consider this test if carcinoma of the prostate a possibility.
- IVU more useful than ultrasound to investigate the urinary tract if stone or carcinoma suspected, or if chronic UTI suspected.
- Terminal stream urine: for schistosomiasis.
- Cystoscopy: may be required in secondary care to confirm and treat stone or tumour.

TOP TIPS

- The man who has symptoms suggesting cystitis but who has sterile pyuria on MSU probably has urethritis.
- GUM clinics are organised to undertake full investigation, counselling and contact tracing. Referral is essential if STD is likely.
- Prostatitis is often forgotten as a diagnosis – but is very difficult to diagnose with certainty, especially when chronic. A trial of a prolonged course of antibiotics may be justified.
- Painful intercourse – usually a sudden pain – accompanied by bleeding suggests a torn frenulum. This often occurs in a younger man who is frequently very alarmed by the event. Reassure him explaining that this is not sinister and is easily treatable.

- Pain after micturition suggests cystitis. This is unusual in men, and further investigation is indicated if recurrent.
- Intermittent pain with passage of blood clots interspersed with painless haematuria suggests a carcinoma (bladder, ureter (rare) or kidney).
- Remember that candidal balanitis may be the first sign of diabetes.
- Refer the elderly man with an adherent foreskin and balanitis. There could be an underlying carcinoma.

NOTES:

PENILE ULCERATION/ SORES

The GP overview

Presentation of this symptom is nearly always accompanied by fear of sexually transmitted disease, even in elderly or no longer sexually active men. There are a number of other causes, many of which are significant and require investigation.

Differential diagnosis

COMMON
- herpes simplex virus (HSV)
- boil/infected sebaceous cyst
- balanitis: bacterial or fungal
- trauma: zipper injury commonest; also torn frenulum, bites, self-mutilation
- balanitis xerotica obliterans (BXO)

OCCASIONAL
- herpes zoster
- Reiter's syndrome: circinate balanitis
- allergic contact eczema
- chancroid (soft sore: *Haemophilus ducreyi*)
- granuloma inguinale (*Klebsiella granulomatis*: tropical infection)
- lymphogranuloma venereum (tropical infection)

RARE
- syphilis (chancre)
- carcinoma of the penis
- tuberculosis
- dermatological conditions, e.g. Behçet's syndrome, lichen planus
- fixed drug eruption

Ready reckoner

	Herpes simplex	Boil	Balanitis	Trauma	BXO
Dysuria	Possible	No	Possible	Possible	Possible
Contact with symptoms	Possible	No	Possible	No	No
Inguinal nodes enlarged	Yes	Possible	Possible	No	No
Discrete single lesion	No	Yes	No	Possible	No
Generally unwell	Possible	No	No	No	No

Possible investigations

LIKELY: swab, syphilis serology.

POSSIBLE: urinalysis, FBC, ESR/CRP.

SMALL PRINT: patch testing, biopsy.

- Urinalysis: in balanitis, may detect undiagnosed diabetes.
- Swab: may reveal infectious cause, e.g. herpes simplex, *Candida*, chancroid, lymphogranuloma venereum and granuloma inguinale (if STD suspected, then other appropriate swabs and blood tests for coexistent disease will be performed at GUM clinic).
- FBC and ESR/CRP: raised WCC and ESR/CRP in significant infection or inflammation (e.g. Reiter's syndrome).
- Syphilis serology: if syphilis suspected (*Note:* may take up to 3 months to become positive after initial infection).
- Patch testing: if allergic contact eczema a possibility.
- Biopsy (in secondary care): to confirm suspected malignancy or reveal underlying skin condition (e.g. lichen planus).

TOP TIPS

- Take a full sexual history, even in the older patient. If STD is suspected, refer to a GUM clinic for investigation, counselling and contact tracing.
- A diagnosis of HSV may induce a number of worries in the patient, some of them well founded, others less so. Give the patient plenty of time to talk through the diagnosis and its implications properly.
- Whatever the cause, the patient is very likely to fear a STD. Ensure that inappropriate anxieties are resolved.
- Enquire after coexistent or previous dermatological problems in obscure cases – this may provide the diagnosis (e.g. lichen planus).

- ☑ A history of travel or sexual contact with travellers is important: a number of the more obscure causes are 'tropical'.
- ☑ Take a sexual history: syphilis is rare generally but is more common in homosexuals.
- ☑ Balanitis and urethritis, arthritis and conjunctivitis form the triad of Reiter's syndrome. Always make a thorough general systemic enquiry.
- ☑ A single, unexplained, persistent ulcer needs thorough investigation as significant disease (infection or malignancy) is likely.
- ☑ Remember the possibility of underlying diabetes in severe or recurrent candidal balanitis.

NOTES:

SCROTAL SWELLING

The GP overview

Scrotal swellings can occur at any age. They arise most commonly from the testicle and its coverings, the spermatic cord and the skin. Greater awareness of testicular cancer has resulted in increasing numbers of young men attending the GP, usually with benign lumps.

Differential diagnosis

COMMON
- inguinal hernia
- sebaceous cyst
- hydrocoele
- epididymal cyst
- epididymo-orchitis (EO)

OCCASIONAL
- torsion of the testis
- iatrogenic sepsis: surgery and catheterisation
- haematocoele
- varicocoele
- congestive heart failure
- post-vasectomy swelling (aseptic), including haematoma, inflammatory reaction to spilt sperm
- trauma – haematoma

RARE
- testicular tumour (seminoma, teratoma)
- ascites
- inferior vena caval thrombosis
- tuberculosis and syphilis (not rare abroad)
- elephantiasis (filariasis)

Ready reckoner

	Hernia	Sebaceous cyst	Hydrocoele	Epididymal cyst	EO
Can get above swelling	No	Yes	Yes	Yes	Yes
Testicle tender	No	No	No	Possible	Yes
Swelling fixed to skin	No	Yes	No	No	No
Tender groin nodes	No	Possible	No	No	Possible
Transilluminates	No	No	Yes	Possible	No

Possible investigations

LIKELY: none.

POSSIBLE: urinalysis, MSU, ultrasound.

SMALL PRINT: FBC, U&E, LFT, CXR, urethral swab, AFP and β-HCG.

- Urinalysis may show signs of UTI, but may be negative in epididymo-orchitis, as may MSU.
- If urethra discharging take urethral swab for gonococcus and *Chlamydia*.
- Ultrasound useful to distinguish solid from cystic swelling.
- FBC, AFP and β-HCG essential baseline investigations if solid tumour suspected – would be arranged by the specialist after referral.
- CXR may show cannonball metastases if carcinoma has spread.
- May require further investigations such as U&E, LFT, syphilis serology if underlying pathology (e.g. ascites, cardiac failure, syphilis) suspected.

TOP TIPS

- Don't forget that the patient's main fear is likely to be cancer. Broach this even if the swelling is obviously benign.
- Examine the patient standing. Many lumps are easier to feel this way and some – especially varicocoeles – may disappear on lying down.
- In the older patient, with bilateral swelling, there is likely to be some underlying disease process such as cardiac failure.
- Consider arranging an ultrasound if a patient remains very anxious about an obviously cystic swelling, or if you have any doubt yourself – a normal result will relieve both parties.

☑ Seminoma may often feel smooth and mimic a large normal testis. Do not rely on the absence of clinical features of malignancy – if the patient feels there has been a change in the testis, act on it.

☑ It can be difficult to distinguish between hernias and hydrocoeles in babies. Hernias require surgical attention; hydrocoeles may resolve within the first year of life. If in doubt, refer.

☑ Remember that a hydrocoele may be caused by an underlying malignancy; in younger patients, always refer, while in the elderly, examine the testis carefully after aspiration.

☑ Left supraclavicular nodes may be involved after tumour spread to para-aortic nodes (can be massive). Examine the abdomen and chest if any suspicion of malignancy.

☑ If any suspicion of torsion – admit urgently.

NOTES:

TESTICULAR PAIN

The GP overview

This is an uncommon symptom in everyday general practice. Though commonest in the young adult, it can affect all age groups. In its acute form, it is excruciating and disabling. In the chronic form it is usually described as a dull ache or dragging sensation. It is the former which causes the GP the most diagnostic difficulty and anxiety.

Differential diagnosis

COMMON
- acute orchitis (mumps, and less commonly scarlet fever and flu)
- acute epididymo-orchitis (EO) (UTI and sexually transmitted infection)
- torsion of the testis
- epididymal cyst
- referred from ureteric stone

OCCASIONAL
- varicocoele
- haematocoele
- hydrocoele
- trauma (fractured testis)
- undescended or misplaced testis
- torsion of the appendix testis
- post-vasectomy pain
- idiopathic chronic testicular pain (accounts for 25% of chronic cases)

RARE
- testicular carcinoma (teratoma and seminoma)
- incarcerated or strangulated inguinoscrotal hernia
- syphilis
- referred from spinal tumours
- neuralgia testis
- tuberculosis of the testis

Ready reckoner

	Orchitis	EO	Torsion	Epididymal cyst	Stone
Testicle tender	Yes	Yes	Yes	No	No
Urethral discharge	No	Possible	No	No	No
Fever	Yes	Possible	No	No	No
Testis high in scrotum	No	No	Yes	No	No
Transilluminating lump	No	No	No	Yes	No

Possible investigations

LIKELY: urinalysis, MSU.

POSSIBLE: urethral swab, ultrasound.

SMALL PRINT: lumbosacral spine and abdominal X-rays, syphilis serology.

- Urinalysis: protein, blood and pus cells in EO. Blood alone with stone.
- MSU: will identify UTI.
- Urethral swab for gonococcus and *Chlamydia* necessary if STD suspected.
- Plain lumbosacral spine and abdominal X-rays are valuable to investigate referred testicular pain (stones and spinal pathology).
- Ultrasound is good at 'seeing' if a testicular mass arises from the body of the testis or its coverings, and whether solid or not.
- Syphilis serology: if syphilis suspected.

TOP TIPS

- In an adult, relief of pain by elevating the testicle suggests epididymitis.
- A negative urinalysis does not exclude epididymitis.
- In mild, chronic testicular ache, examine the patient standing up, otherwise you may miss a varicocoele.

- A sudden onset of excruciating pain associated with nausea suggests torsion of testis – especially in children and adolescents. Admit immediately.
- Repeated episodes of spontaneously resolving pain may represent recurrent, self-correcting torsion. Refer for possible orchidopexy and warn the patient to report urgently if there is severe and persisting pain.
- If non-gonococcal/chlamydial epididymitis is clinically suspected, treat immediately with a broad-spectrum antibiotic.
- If epididymitis does not settle with antibiotics, consider abscess formation – admit for IV antibiotics or surgical drainage.

VAGINAL DISCHARGE

The GP overview

Vaginal discharge is usually a symptom of the reproductive years, but can occur at any age. It can be influenced by the menstrual cycle, use of 'the pill', age, pregnancy and sexual activity. Treatment is often simple, but if it fails, or if there are risk factors for STDs, it is sensible to refer to a GUM clinic.

Differential diagnosis

COMMON
- excessive normal secretions
- thrush
- bacterial vaginosis (BV)
- trichomonal vaginosis (TV)
- cervicitis (gonococcus, *Chlamydia*, herpes)

OCCASIONAL
- cervical ectropion
- cervical polyp
- lost tampon, ring pessary or other foreign body
- IUCD
- bartholinitis
- salpingitis

RARE
- vulvovaginal neoplasia
- cervical or uterine neoplasia
- sloughing intrauterine fibroid
- pyometra
- pelvic fistula

Ready reckoner

	Normal	Thrush	BV	TV	Cervicitis
Intense itch	No	Yes	No	Possible	Possible
Offensive smell	No	No	Yes	Yes	Possible
Vulval soreness	No	Yes	No	Yes	Possible
Yellow/green/grey (mucopurulent) discharge	No	No	Yes	Yes	Yes
Inflamed cervix	No	No	No	Yes	Yes

Possible investigations

LIKELY: high vaginal swab (HVS).

POSSIBLE: endocervical swab, urethral swab, urine testing for *Chlamydia*, blood sugar or HbA1c.

SMALL PRINT: other specialist investigations.

Most GPs would confine themselves to the HVS, endocervical swab and urine test. Those with a special interest might undertake the microscopy themselves.

- HVS is simple and readily detects *Candida*, BV and TV.
- Wet saline microscopy shows clue cells in BV, motile trichomonads in TV.
- Gram stain of cervical or urethral exudate shows negatively staining diplococci in up to 85% of gonococcal infections.
- Endocervical swab for ELISA is the gold standard for detecting *Chlamydia*.
- DNA amplification testing of first-catch urine (not MSU) specimens for *Chlamydia* is non-invasive and relatively acceptable to patients.
- Blood sugar or HbA1c: to detect diabetes in severe or recurrent thrush.
- Specialist investigations might include D&C or hysteroscopy (for possible malignancy) and barium enema (for pelvic fistula).

TOP TIPS

- It is reasonable to diagnose and treat thrush empirically in a woman with classical symptoms who has had the problem before – many women successfully self-medicate and only attend to obtain their treatment free, via a prescription. But if in any doubt about the diagnosis, examine and investigate as appropriate.
- It is worth investing time with the patient suffering confirmed recurrent thrush – advice supplemented by written patient information may help minimise future problems.
- Make sure you have all the appropriate swabs (HVS, endocervical, urethral) to hand – you never know when you might need them.
- Excessive concern about normal secretions might mask a sexual problem or worry – enquire discreetly about this.

- Recurrent or florid thrush may be a presentation of undiagnosed diabetes mellitus. Ask about thirst, polyuria and tiredness and check a fasting glucose if any suspicion of underlying diabetes, or there is a positive family history of diabetes.
- Vaginal discharge is an uncommon symptom before puberty. Don't forget the possibilities of abuse or a foreign body.
- Always conduct a full pelvic examination in the post-menopausal woman with vaginal discharge. Malignancy is one of the likeliest causes.
- A florid erosion is likely to be caused by chlamydial cervicitis – take a swab and treat appropriately.
- If you suspect a sexually transmitted disease, refer to the GUM clinic for full assessment and contact tracing. Refer urgently to the GUM clinic or duty gynaecologist if there are systemic flu-like symptoms and fever with pelvic pain and vaginal discharge.

NOTES:

VULVAL IRRITATION

The GP overview

Vulval irritation encompasses soreness and itch and is a very common presentation in primary care. Embarrassment may mean a 'calling card' symptom has first to be presented. Sometimes it is a 'calling card' itself, being easier to talk about than a psychosexual problem. With sensitivity, the real issues should emerge during the consultation.

Differential diagnosis

COMMON
- thrush: *Candida* infection
- *Trichomonas vaginalis*
- chemical: bubble baths, detergents, 'feminine hygiene' douches
- trauma: insufficient lubrication during intercourse
- atrophic vaginitis

OCCASIONAL
- ammoniacal vulvitis from incontinence
- skin disorders (e.g. eczema, psoriasis, lichen planus)
- infestations: threadworms, pubic lice
- psychosexual problems
- other infections (e.g. genital warts or herpes)

RARE
- diabetes (without *Candida* infection)
- vulval dysplasia (various other terms for this include lichen sclerosis et atrophicus, leukoplakia)
- vulval carcinoma
- general disorder causing pruritus (e.g. jaundice, leukaemia, chronic renal failure, lymphoma)
- psychogenic (no organic or psychosexual problem)

Ready reckoner

	Thrush	Trichomonas	Chemical	Trauma	Atrophic vaginitis
Itching prominent	Yes	Possible	Yes	Possible	No
Soreness prominent	Possible	Yes	Yes	Yes	Yes
White discharge	Yes	No	No	No	No
Fishy, smelly discharge	No	Yes	No	No	No
Thin, dry, red mucosa	No	No	No	No	Yes

Possible investigations

LIKELY: HVS (if discharge present).

POSSIBLE: urinalysis.

SMALL PRINT: FBC, LFT, U&E, fasting sugar or HbA1c, vulval biopsy.

- Urinalysis for sugar: diabetes predisposes to thrush and glycosuria in itself can cause vulvitis.
- FBC, LFT, U&E: if vulvitis is part of a generalised pruritus, or if the patient is generally unwell, these blood tests may reveal blood dyscrasias or renal or hepatic dysfunction.
- Fasting sugar or HbA1c to diagnose or rule out underlying diabetes.
- HVS: identifying the pathogen if discharge is present will help management in puzzling or recurrent cases.
- Vulval biopsy (secondary care): multiple biopsies are required if vulval dysplasia or carcinoma are suspected.

TOP TIPS

- It is easy to make an erroneous diagnosis of UTI in a patient with vulvitis: external dysuria and contamination of urine with pus cells and blood (especially if there is an associated discharge) may mislead the unwary. Helpful pointers are the presence of external vulval irritation and the absence of frequency or urgency.
- In obscure cases, check the skin elsewhere. Vulval irritation may be a manifestation of a primary skin disorder, such as eczema or psoriasis.
- The aetiology may be multifactorial with, for example, some primary cause leading to secondary chemical irritation from over-washing or the use of douches. A careful history is needed to unravel the underlying cause and exacerbating factors.
- Recurrent candidal infection is a particular problem. Various therapeutic strategies are available, but it is important to take time to explore the woman's perception of the cause, explain the diagnosis and resolve any exacerbating factors.

☑ Post-menopausal atrophic vaginitis causes soreness rather than itch. Dysplasias and some carcinomas produce intense irritation. Examine these patients and, if in doubt, refer for biopsy.

☑ Consider diabetes in florid or refractory cases of *Candida* infection.

☑ Significant psychosexual problems may present with vulval irritation. Adopt a sympathetic, open approach. Take particular note of any comments made during the physical examination as this sometimes prompts the patient to reveal the true problem.

☑ Persistent vulval irritation may rarely be a symptom of significant systemic disease. Consider this if the patient has generalised pruritus elsewhere and seems unwell in herself.

☑ If the cause is sexually transmitted (e.g. genital herpes or warts), exclude other infections by referring to a GUM clinic.

NOTES:

VULVAL SWELLING

The GP overview

Vulval swellings may originate in the vulva, or appear there after displacement from their origin. They often present as 'a lump down below' – an expression which belies the variety of possible causes. They generate a lot of anxiety but are rarely sinister.

Differential diagnosis

COMMON
- boils
- sebaceous cysts
- viral warts (condylomata acuminata)
- Bartholin's cyst
- inguinal hernia (may extend down to labium major)

OCCASIONAL
- varicose vein, varicocoele of vulva
- Bartholin's abscess (infected Bartholin's cyst)
- fibroma, lipoma, hidradenoma
- uterine prolapse, cystocoele, rectocoele, enterocoele (hernia of the pouch of Douglas)
- urethral caruncle (meatal prolapse)

RARE
- cervical polyp
- carcinoma (95% are squamous)
- endometrioma
- hydrocoele of the canal of Nuck
- traumatic haematoma

Ready reckoner

	Boil	Sebaceous cyst	Viral warts	Bartholin's cyst	Inguinal hernia
Tender	Yes	No	No	No	No
Reducible	No	No	No	No	Yes
Multiple	Possible	Possible	Yes	No	No
Epidermal	Yes	Yes	Yes	No	No
Central punctum	No	Yes	No	No	No

Possible investigations

There are no investigations likely to be performed in primary care: the diagnosis is almost always established by history and examination. If it isn't, then referral is usually required.

TOP TIPS

◩ Remember that, to many patients, a lump means cancer until proven otherwise. You may only require a cursory glance to reassure yourself that the problem is insignificant – but the patient may interpret your approach as dismissive or inadequate. Ensure that the patient's anxieties are resolved by adequate examination and explanation.

◩ If the lump is not obviously apparent, or is poorly defined, examine the patient standing: this may reveal a hernia, varicocoele or prolapse.

◩ A varicocoele of the vulva has a characteristic 'bag of worms' feel. It often appears and gets worse during pregnancy.

◩ A persistent, ulcerating lump in the vulva must always be referred for biopsy to exclude carcinoma, even though some benign lumps can ulcerate (e.g. hidradenoma).

◩ Check for lymphadenopathy: hard inguinal nodes with a painless lump are highly suggestive of malignancy. The lump can occasionally be a metastasis itself.

◩ Women with genital warts may have coexisting sexually transmitted infection: refer to the local GUM clinic for appropriate investigation and, if necessary, contact tracing.

NOTES:

VULVAL ULCERATION/ SORES

The GP overview

This often unpleasant symptom is uncommon, but very important, as many causes are significant and require specialist investigation, treatment and follow-up. Patients often have difficulty visualising or describing these types of lesions, so adequate examination is vital in establishing the diagnosis.

Differential diagnosis

COMMON
- herpes simplex virus (HSV)
- thrush (particularly if very excoriated)
- vulval dysplasia
- squamous cell carcinoma (SCC): 95% of vulval malignancies
- excoriated scabies

OCCASIONAL
- allergic contact eczema
- chancroid: *H. ducreyi* (tropical)
- granuloma inguinale: *K. granulomatis* (tropical)
- lymphogranuloma venereum: *Chlamydia trachomatis* (tropical)
- other malignancies (e.g. BCC, melanoma, adenocarcinoma, sarcoma)
- herpes zoster

RARE
- syphilis and yaws
- Behçet's syndrome
- tuberculosis
- fixed drug eruption
- dermatological disorders (e.g. pemphigus and pemphigoid)

Ready reckoner

	HSV	Thrush	Vulval dysplasia	SCC	Excoriated scabies
Fever, malaise	Yes	No	No	No	No
Prodromal tingling	Yes	No	No	No	No
Itchy	No	Yes	Yes	Possible	Yes
Vaginal discharge	Possible	Yes	No	No	No
Inguinal lymphadenopathy	Yes	No	No	Possible	No

Possible investigations

LIKELY: urinalysis, swab.

POSSIBLE: fasting sugar or HbA1c, and (in secondary care) biopsy.

SMALL PRINT: syphilis serology, patch testing.

- ▧ Urinalysis: glycosuria may be present in undiagnosed diabetes presenting with severe or recurrent *Candida* infection. Fasting sugar or HbA1c to rule out or diagnose undiagnosed diabetes.
- ▧ Swab for microscopy and culture: may help in the diagnosis of various infections such as HSV, *Candida*, chancroid, granuloma inguinale and lymphogranuloma venereum (if STD suspected, then other relevant swabs and blood tests for coexistent infection will be performed at GUM clinic).
- ▧ Syphilis serology: if syphilis a possibility (*Note:* serology may not become positive for up to 3 months after infection).
- ▧ Patch testing: may help in the diagnosis of allergic contact eczema.
- ▧ Biopsy (in secondary care): for any persistent ulcer to confirm diagnosis – may reveal carcinoma, vulval dysplasia or underlying skin disorder.

TOP TIPS

- ▧ A diagnosis of HSV can be traumatic for a woman. Spend time discussing the nature of the problem and its recurrent nature, including implications for sexual partners and future pregnancies.
- ▧ If the patient suffers recurrent vulval ulceration, offer to see her as an 'urgent' during the next attack to visualise the lesions and arrange microbiological testing.
- ▧ In obscure cases do not confine the history and examination to the vulva. Lesions elsewhere (e.g. with pemphigus or Behçet's syndrome) may give the clue needed to make the diagnosis.

☑ History of travel and sexual contact with travellers is very important as there are a number of 'tropical' causes.

☑ The more straightforward causes (HSV and severe excoriated thrush) usually result in multiple ulcers, with the diagnosis being obvious from the history and examination. Take very seriously any single persistent vulval sore: significant disease is likely.

☑ If you suspect a sexually transmitted disease, refer urgently to the local GUM clinic for appropriate investigations and contact tracing.

☑ Remember the possibility of undiagnosed diabetes in severe *Candida* infection.

☑ The pregnant woman near term with primary HSV is in danger of transmitting the virus to her newborn – a situation with a significant mortality and morbidity. Contact the obstetrician urgently to arrange probable elective Caesarian section.

NOTES:

HAIR AND NAILS

Abnormal nails

Excess body hair

Hair loss

Itchy scalp

ABNORMAL NAILS

The GP overview

Women are far more likely to present with this symptom than men, often for cosmetic reasons. The likeliest queries relate to normal nails that break easily or are not smooth. Other abnormalities may be detected during physical examination rather than being volunteered by the patient, and may indicate significant pathology.

Differential diagnosis

COMMON

- psoriasis
- fungal infection: onychomycosis
- trauma to nail bed
- trauma due to biting (also hang nail)
- onychogryphosis (OG)

OCCASIONAL

- trophic changes (Beau's lines) – appear 2–3 months after severe illness
- hand eczema
- longitudinal ridging (onychorrhexis)
- chronic paronychia
- clubbing (various causes)
- autoimmune disease (e.g. alopecia areata, lichen planus)
- koilonychia (spoon nails): iron deficiency anaemia and Plummer–Vinson syndrome

RARE

- subungual melanoma
- leuconychia (e.g. liver disease, diabetes)
- lamellar nail dystrophy
- yellow nail syndrome (may be accompanied by chronic bronchitis, bronchiectasis or pleural effusion)
- exfoliative dermatitis: nail shedding
- nail dystrophy due to poor circulation (e.g. Raynaud's disease)
- epidermolysis bullosa

Ready reckoner

	Trauma	Psoriasis	Fungal	Biting	OG
Pitting on nails	No	Yes	No	No	No
Nails symmetrically affected	No	Yes	No	Possible	No
Ragged edges	No	No	No	Yes	No
Increased thickness	Possible	Possible	Yes	No	Yes
Friable and crumbly	No	Possible	Yes	No	No

Possible investigations

LIKELY: nail clippings for mycology.

POSSIBLE: urinalysis, FBC.

SMALL PRINT: LFT, CXR.

- ◪ Nail clippings for mycology may be the only way to differentiate psoriatic nail dystrophy and onychomycosis.
- ◪ Urinalysis worthwhile if nails are unusually white: this can occur in diabetes.
- ◪ FBC may confirm iron deficiency anaemia in koilonychia.
- ◪ LFT: to assess liver function in leuconychia.
- ◪ CXR worthwhile if chest symptoms with clubbing or yellow nails.

TOP TIPS

- ◪ Don't confine your examination to the nails – useful clues may be found elsewhere, e.g. patches of psoriasis or coexisting tinea corporis.
- ◪ The commonest differentials are psoriasis and fungal infections. The latter are usually asymmetrical.
- ◪ Patients usually worry about vitamin or calcium deficiencies – these are never the real cause.
- ◪ By the time Beau's lines are obvious to the patient, 3 months or so will have passed from the precipitating event – look back in the records for aetiological clues.

- ◪ Subungual melanoma is rare and is easily confused with the much more common subungual haematoma. Possible pointers include nail destruction, extension of pigment onto the nail fold and longitudinal bands of pigment. If in doubt, refer.
- ◪ Clubbing is really an abnormality of the fingertips; if noted, be alert to signs of major pulmonary or cardiac disease. Carcinoma of the lung is the commonest cause.
- ◪ Don't assume crumbly white nails are caused by fungus. Before embarking on lengthy antifungal treatment, try to confirm the diagnosis with nail clippings.
- ◪ Severely bitten nails may be a minor symptom of a major anxiety disorder. Be aware of the possible need to explore psychological issues.

EXCESS BODY HAIR

The GP overview

This is defined as excess growth of terminal hair in women in male distribution sites (i.e. chin, cheeks, upper lip, lower abdomen and thighs). It presents as a cosmetic problem. Ethnic origin must be taken into account: Mediterraneans and Indians grow more than Nordics. Japanese, Chinese and American Indians grow the least. In the UK, according to surveys, up to 15% of women believe they have excess body hair, although only a minority present to the GP.

Differential diagnosis

COMMON
- constitutional (physiological)
- polycystic ovary syndrome (PCOS): 50% of cases
- anorexia nervosa
- menopause
- iatrogenic, e.g. phenytoin, minoxidil, danazol, glucocorticoids

OCCASIONAL
- congenital adrenal hyperplasia (1 in 5000)
- anabolic steroid abuse
- ovarian tumours: arrhenoblastoma, hilus cell tumour, luteoma
- adrenal tumours: carcinoma and adenoma
- congenital (1 in 5000 live births) and juvenile hypothyroidism

RARE
- acromegaly (incidence 3 per million)
- porphyria cutanea tarda
- Cushing's syndrome (incidence 1–2 per million)
- hypertrichosis lanuginosa
- Cornelia de Lange syndrome (Amsterdam dwarfism)

Ready reckoner

	Constitutional	PCOS	Anorexia	Menopause	Drugs
Excess vellous hair	No	No	Yes	No	Possible
Facial hirsutism	Possible	Possible	No	Yes	Possible
Oligo/amenorrhoea	No	Yes	Yes	Yes	No
Otherwise well	Yes	Yes	No	Possible	Possible
Weight loss	No	No	Yes	No	No

Possible investigations

LIKELY: none.

POSSIBLE: serum testosterone, pelvic ultrasound, FBC, U&E, TFT.

SMALL PRINT: FSH/LH, other tests of endocrine function and specialised imaging techniques (for adrenal/pituitary disorders), urinary porphyrins.

- ☑ Serum testosterone: probably the most useful investigation. Mild elevation (up to three times the normal value) suggests PCOS; levels above this indicate a possible tumour.
- ☑ FBC, U&E: possible iron deficiency anaemia and electrolyte disturbance in anorexia; U&E may be deranged in adrenal disorders.
- ☑ FSH/LH and TFT: the former may help to confirm menopause and may point towards PCOS (elevated LH, normal FSH); the latter reveals hypothyroidism.
- ☑ Other tests of endocrine function and imaging techniques: to investigate possible adrenal and pituitary disorders (usually undertaken in secondary care).
- ☑ Pelvic ultrasound: multiple ovarian cysts characteristic of PCOS; may also reveal ovarian tumour.
- ☑ Urinary porphyrins: for porphyria.

TOP TIPS

- ☑ Mild, long-standing hirsutism does not require investigation.
- ☑ Enquire about self-medication, especially in athletes – anabolic steroids may occasionally be the cause.
- ☑ Take the problem seriously and be prepared for questions about cosmetic treatments such as bleaching, depilatory creams and electrolysis.

- Sudden and severe hirsutism is the most important marker for serious underlying pathology.
- Other clues suggesting a possible hormone-secreting tumour include amenorrhoea, onset of baldness at the same time as hirsutism and a patient who seems generally unwell.
- Consider psychological factors: hirsutism can cause – or be the presenting complaint in – significant depression.
- Recent onset of significant headache and visual field defect raise the possibility of a pituitary adenoma.

NOTES:

HAIR LOSS

The GP overview

A distressing symptom for both genders: men fear loss of potency, and women are horrified at the cosmetic disaster unfolding. The psychological significance of increased hairfall is all too easy to overlook in a typical busy surgery. Take care to acknowledge that the problem is being taken seriously.

Differential diagnosis

COMMON
- androgenic alopecia (male pattern baldness)
- seborrhoeic dermatitis
- alopecia areata
- contact allergic dermatitis
- tinea capitis

OCCASIONAL
- bacterial folliculitis
- telogen effluvium
- endocrine: myxoedema, hypopituitarism and hypoparathyroidism
- traction alopecia
- lupus erythematosus

RARE
- secondary syphilis
- trichotillomania
- morphoea
- iatrogenic, e.g. chemotherapy, anticoagulants
- malnutrition

Ready reckoner

	Androgenic	Seborrhoeic dermatitis	Alopecia areata	Allergic dermatitis	Tinea capitis
Normal scalp	Yes	No	Yes	No	No
Abnormal skin on body	No	Possible	No	Possible	Possible
Exclamation mark hairs	No	No	Yes	No	No
Patchy hair thinning	Yes (M)	Yes	Yes	Yes	Yes
	No (F)				
Scaling and weeping	No	Yes	No	Possible	Yes

Possible investigations

LIKELY: none.

POSSIBLE: Wood's light test, hair and scales for mycology.

SMALL PRINT: FBC, ESR/CRP, U&E, TFT, FSH/LH, prolactin, autoimmune tests, syphilis serology.

- *Microsporum* infections will fluoresce green under a Wood's (UV) light.
- Send scrapings and hair for mycology if the scalp looks abnormal.
- FBC, ESR/CRP and autoimmune tests may help identify autoimmune causes, e.g. SLE.
- Syphilis serology: old-fashioned, but syphilis is on the increase.
- U&E, TFT, FSH/LH/prolactin will effectively screen for endocrinopathy.

TOP TIPS

- Alopecia areata is occasionally associated with other autoimmune diseases. Further assessment is sensible, even at a later consultation.
- Remember that in telogen effluvium, the traumatic event – such as a significant illness or childbirth – will have taken place about 4 months before the onset of hair loss, so the connection is unlikely to be made by the patient.
- The patient invariably fears total hair loss – ensure that this is broached and that a realistic prognosis is given.
- Reassure men with male-pattern baldness who are anxious about their potency. In this case it signifies the opposite. Its onset is related to adequate circulating testosterone. Eunuchs tend not to go bald.
- Lymphadenopathy in association with alopecia may suggest an infective process: consider bacterial folliculitis.

- Alopecia areata has a particularly poor prognosis if there are several patches, there is loss of eyebrows or eyelashes, or if it begins in childhood.
- Scarring alopecia should prompt the clinician to look for general signs of lupus erythematosus.
- Trichotillomania in children is usually simply due to habit; in adults, though, it is more often a sign of significant psychological disturbance.

NOTES:

ITCHY SCALP

The GP overview

This might appear a mundane symptom to the GP, but it can cause the patient significant distress. It's usually a welcome presentation, as it's perceived as a quickie – one of those problems in which a brief examination can be performed at the same time as an equally brief history. This approach generally pays dividends, but the problem can sometimes be more complicated than it might at first appear.

Differential diagnosis

COMMON
- head lice
- seborrhoeic eczema
- psoriasis
- lichen simplex
- impetigo (may be underlying head lice or eczema)

OCCASIONAL
- allergic/contact eczema
- other fungal infections

RARE
- stress/depression
- viral infection, e.g. chickenpox – a common problem but only rarely presents with scalp itch

Ready reckoner

	Head lice	Seborrhoeic eczema	Psoriasis	Lichen simplex	Impetigo
Scaly scalp	No	Yes	Yes	Possible	No
Pustular lesions	Possible	No	No	No	Yes
Skin lesions elsewhere	No	Possible	Possible	Possible	Possible
Visible egg cases	Yes	No	No	No	No
Chronic problem	No	Possible	Yes	Possible	No

Possible investigations

It is highly unlikely that any investigations will be required at all. Confirmation of a fungal infection may be obtained via fluorescence under a Wood's light or by microscopy and culture of scalp and hair samples.

TOP TIPS

- Whatever the actual diagnosis, scratching will perpetuate or complicate the problem and so should be discouraged.
- Consider examining the skin and nails, as these may provide useful additional clues.
- The diagnosis in a child is very likely to be head lice; the list of differentials increases the older the patient.

- Scalp impetigo in a child – particularly if it relapses rapidly – suggests an underlying problem such as head lice or eczema. This needs treating too, or the symptom will persist.
- In an otherwise puzzling case, consider psychological causes – stress and depression can sometimes present with scalp itching.

NOTES:

LIMBS

Acute single joint pain

Arm and shoulder pain

Calf pain

Foot pain

Hand and wrist pain

Leg ulcers

Multiple joint pain

Painful muscles

Recurrent hip area pain in an adult

Recurrent knee pain

Swollen ankles

Swollen calf

ACUTE SINGLE JOINT PAIN

The GP overview

This is a very common problem in primary care. Usually, there are few physical signs, although occasionally a genuine monoarthritis with all the classical signs of inflammation will present. Overall, the most likely aetiological factor is trauma, though other conditions may already affect a joint. In the elderly, an exacerbation of osteoarthritis is common; this condition may also cause multiple joint pain. The knee is probably the single most frequently affected joint.

Differential diagnosis

COMMON
- ◩ acute exacerbation of osteoarthritis (OA)
- ◩ traumatic synovitis
- ◩ gout/pseudogout
- ◩ chondromalacia patellae (CP) and other anterior knee pain syndromes
- ◩ traumatic haemarthrosis (e.g. after cruciate ligament injury)

OCCASIONAL
- ◩ fracture
- ◩ Reiter's disease
- ◩ psoriatic arthritis
- ◩ rheumatoid arthritis (RA)
- ◩ patellar tendinitis, Osgood–Schlatter's disease

RARE
- ◩ septic arthritis (SA)
- ◩ haemophilia
- ◩ local tropical infections (e.g. Madura foot (mycetoma pedis), filariasis)
- ◩ malignancy (usually secondary)
- ◩ avascular necrosis
- ◩ recurrent joint subluxation

Ready reckoner

	OA	CP/anterior knee pain	Synovitis	Gout	Traumatic haemarthrosis
Sudden onset	Possible	No	Yes	Possible	Yes
History of acute trauma	Possible	No	Yes	Possible	Yes
Recurrent problem	Yes	Yes	No	Yes	No
Several joints painful	Possible	No	No	Possible	No
Hot, red joint	No	No	No	Yes	Possible

Possible investigations

LIKELY: none.

POSSIBLE: FBC, ESR/CRP, uric acid, X-ray, joint aspiration (in monoarthritis of large joint).

SMALL PRINT: rheumatoid factor, clotting studies/factor VIII assay, arthroscopy.

◪ FBC/ESR/CRP: WCC and ESR/CRP raised in infection, systemic inflammatory conditions; Hb may be reduced in the latter.

◪ Uric acid: once attack has subsided, useful to add weight to clinical diagnosis of gout (especially if considering treatment with allopurinol).

◪ Rheumatoid factor may be useful if symptoms suggest possible RA.

◪ X-ray: essential if fracture suspected. May also reveal OA, avascular necrosis, malignancy and help to distinguish between RA and psoriatic arthritis.

◪ Sterile aspiration of joint fluid: to look for pus (septic arthritis), blood (haemarthrosis) and crystals (gout/pseudogout).

◪ Clotting studies/factor VIII assay: if haemophilia a possibility.

◪ Arthroscopy: may be required urgently in secondary care if trauma has resulted in a haemarthrosis.

TOP TIPS

◪ Autoimmune blood tests can be misleading in possible arthritis. The diagnosis should be clinical; blood testing simply adds weight and prognostic information to the clinical assessment. Positive tests can be found in normal patients – beware of inappropriately labelling an insignificant problem as a significant arthritis on the basis of a blood test.

◪ Gout is very painful, will limit movement and may cause a slight fever. Septic arthritis gives a similar picture but with marked restriction of movement and, usually, a high fever. If in doubt, arrange urgent assessment.

◪ In obscure cases, question and examine the patient carefully. For example, in Reiter's disease, symptoms of urethritis or conjunctivitis may have been minimal or forgotten; in psoriatic arthritis, there may only be insignificant skin lesions.

☑ If one joint is red, very hot, intensely painful with marked limitation of movement and systemic illness, septic arthritis must be excluded: admit.

☑ Haemarthrosis usually develops rapidly after trauma and indicates significant damage requiring immediate referral; effusion due to synovitis usually takes a day or longer to accumulate and is less urgent.

☑ Septic arthritis is notoriously easy to miss in a patient with coexisting RA. The systemic signs may be absent and the diagnosis may mistakenly be viewed as a flare-up of rheumatoid arthritis.

☑ A young adult male with a monoarthritis of the knee not caused by trauma is likely to have Reiter's disease.

NOTES:

ARM AND SHOULDER PAIN

The GP overview

Arm pain is a common presentation with a wide differential. Many generalised disorders, such as arthritis, neuropathy and polymyalgia, cause widespread symptoms, which may involve the arm – these are not considered here. Instead, this section concentrates on pain specific to the arm, or pain characteristically referred to the arm.

Differential diagnosis

COMMON

- simple muscular strain
- epicondylitis (tennis or golfer's elbow)
- subacromial bursitis/capsulitis
- cervical spondylosis
- angina

OCCASIONAL

- bicipital tendonitis
- acromioclavicular and sternoclavicular joint pain
- acute calcific tendonitis
- de Quervain's tenosynovitis
- carpal tunnel (CT) syndrome
- cervical rib
- brachial and ulnar neuritis (including post-herpetic pain)
- cervical and thoracic disc prolapse

RARE

- GORD
- malignancy: local bone cancer, spinal cord, spine and lung
- subclavian aneurysm
- multiple sclerosis
- syphilitic aortitis
- thoracic outlet syndrome

Ready reckoner

	Epicondylitis	Muscle strain	Cervical spondylosis	Bursitis/ capsulitis	Angina
Worse moving arm/hand	Yes	Yes	Possible	Yes	No
Hand paraesthesiae	No	No	Possible	No	Possible
Exercise related	Possible	Possible	No	Possible	Yes
Local arm tenderness	Yes	Possible	No	Possible	No
Limitation of movement	Possible	Possible	Possible	Yes	No

Possible investigations

LIKELY: none.

POSSIBLE: FBC, ESR/CRP, TFT, ECG/secondary care cardiac investigations, nerve conduction studies, chest and neck X-ray.

SMALL PRINT: other X-rays/bone scan, MRI scan, lumbar puncture, syphilis serology.

▨ FBC, ESR/CRP: may be anaemia and raised ESR/CRP in inflammatory or malignant conditions.

▨ TFT: myxoedema and carpal tunnel syndrome significantly associated.

▨ Neck X-ray sometimes useful to confirm diagnosis of cervical spondylosis and assess its severity – but cervical spondylosis on X-ray does not correlate well with symptoms and may just be an incidental finding.

▨ ECG/secondary care cardiac investigations: to pursue possible diagnosis of angina.

▨ Nerve conduction studies: will help confirm nerve entrapment (e.g. carpal tunnel).

▨ CXR: for apical tumour.

▨ Other X-rays/bone scans: if bony tumour (especially secondaries) suspected. Calcium deposits may be seen in acute calcific tendonitis.

▨ MRI scan, lumbar puncture: if MS suspected; scanning may also be helpful to visualise possible cord lesion (all likely to be arranged after specialist referral).

▨ Syphilis serology: in the rare case of possible syphilis.

TOP TIPS

▨ It is tempting to view arm pain as a welcome 'quickie'; in fact, a careful history is important to exclude the more unusual serious pathologies and the examination should usually serve only to confirm an already formulated diagnosis.

▨ Patients with arm pain – especially if it is accompanied by intermittent paraesthesiae – are often inappropriately concerned that the diagnosis may be angina or a stroke. Make sure these fears are properly explored.

▨ The natural history of many of the more common problems (e.g. subacromial bursitis, epicondylitis) can be quite prolonged. Making this clear from the outset helps maintain the patient's trust in you if the symptoms do take some time to settle.

▱ Getting the patient to indicate the site of pain is a useful ploy in shoulder discomfort. Diffuse pain is typical of capsulitis and subacromial bursitis, whereas, with sternoclavicular or acromioclavicular joint problems, or bicipital tendonitis, the area is more likely to be very localised.

▱ Beware of persistent paraesthesiae with arm pain, especially if the patient also complains of arm or hand weakness; either there is serious nerve compression or some other significant neurological pathology.

▱ Angina may present only with arm pain. Enquire carefully to establish the pattern of the pain.

▱ Apical lung tumour (Pancoast tumour) may cause severe arm pain long before any signs are evident. Investigate smokers with unexplained arm pain.

▱ Consider the other less common diagnoses if the pain is severe and persistent, the diagnosis is not obvious from the history and the patient displays unrestricted arm movements.

NOTES:

CALF PAIN

The GP overview

Calf pain is usually innocent, except when accompanied by swelling. It is often caused by cramp, which is especially common in the elderly. In this group it can cause significant distress, through the havoc wreaked on sleep. Some of the less likely diagnoses, such as peripheral vascular disease, have important implications, so careful assessment is necessary.

Differential diagnosis

COMMON
- idiopathic (simple) cramp (including night cramps)
- muscle stiffness (unaccustomed exercise)
- cellulitis
- peripheral vascular disease (PVD; intermittent claudication)
- muscle injury (e.g. strain)

OCCASIONAL
- referred back pain (L4 and 5)
- referred knee pain (arthropathy, infection)
- alcoholic or diabetic neuropathy
- cramps caused by underlying hypocalcaemia or electrolyte imbalance
- ruptured Baker's cyst
- deep vein thrombosis (DVT)
- thrombophlebitis

RARE
- motor neurone disease
- multiple sclerosis
- muscle enzyme deficiency
- psychological: muscle tension
- lead and strychnine poisoning
- ruptured Achilles tendon

Ready reckoner

	Cramp	Stiffness	Cellulitis	Muscle injury	PVD
Worse at night	Yes	No	No	No	No
Systemically unwell	No	No	Possible	No	No
Worse with exercise	Possible	Yes	Possible	Yes	Yes
Calf swelling	No	No	Yes	Possible	No
Cool peripheries	No	No	No	No	Yes

Possible investigations

LIKELY: none.

POSSIBLE: urinalysis, WCC, ESR/CRP, U&E, LFT, blood glucose or HbA1c, D-dimer.

SMALL PRINT: ultrasound, venogram, angiography.

- Urinalysis: check specific gravity, glucose and protein (over and under-hydration, diabetes, renal failure as occasional causes of 'simple' cramp).
- WCC and ESR/CRP: both raised in infection. ESR/CRP raised in arthropathy.
- U&E and calcium: check renal function and electrolyte imbalance (e.g. from diuretics; hypocalcaemia).
- LFT and blood glucose or HbA1c: if suspect alcoholism or diabetes resulting in a neuropathy.
- D-dimer (usually in hospital): a raised level suggests a DVT, but is not conclusive.
- Consider referring urgently for ultrasound of lower limb veins with or without venography if DVT suspected.
- Angiography will be arranged by the specialist if peripheral vascular disease is suspected.

TOP TIPS

- Save the patient unnecessary investigation and possible anticoagulation by taking a careful history. A muscle tear and a DVT can both produce calf swelling and warmth. The former, though, is preceded by a dramatic and sudden pain in the calf, sometimes described as being like a kick or a gunshot.
- It can be difficult to distinguish a simple muscle strain from claudication. Muscular pains tend to produce discomfort as soon as the patient stands; claudication usually starts after the patient has walked a predictable distance.
- Patients with superficial phlebitis will fear the more serious DVT. Explain the difference to them.
- Do not overlook Achilles rupture. The presentation may sometimes be less dramatic than you would expect.

☑ Children rarely present with cramp (though it is common): avoid labelling as 'growing pains' unless serious causes are excluded.

☑ Consider investigating the adult patient with recent onset of apparently simple cramps if associated with general malaise (these will be in the minority).

☑ Claudication accompanied by nocturnal pain in the ball of the foot suggests critical ischaemia – refer urgently.

☑ Homans's sign is positive in virtually all painful conditions of the calf. It is not diagnostic of DVT.

NOTES:

FOOT PAIN

The GP overview

Pain in the foot is difficult for patients to ignore and so will often present with a relatively short history. Local causes predominate, but remember to think further afield: referral through S1 (lateral border of the foot) and L5 (dorsum of the foot to the big toe) nerve roots may occur. Ankle pain is not considered here.

Differential diagnosis

COMMON
- gout
- verruca
- bunion/hallux valgus
- infected ingrowing toenail (IGTN)
- plantar fasciitis

OCCASIONAL
- Morton's neuroma
- metatarsalgia
- arthritis (osteo and rheumatoid)
- Achilles tendonitis/bursitis
- oedema
- foreign body

RARE
- march fracture
- Sever's disease (apophysitis of the calcaneus), usually a problem of adolescence
- osteochondritis: navicular = Köhler's disease; head of second or third metatarsal = Freiberg's disease
- osteomyelitis and septic arthritis
- erythromelalgia and painful polyneuropathy
- ischaemia

Ready reckoner

	Gout	Verruca	Bunion	IGTN	Plantar fasciitis
Forefoot pain	Yes	Possible	Yes	Yes	No
Very tender joint(s)	Yes	No	Possible	No	No
Pain at rest	Yes	No	No	Possible	No
Tender heel	No	Possible	No	No	Yes
Sudden onset	Yes	No	No	Possible	Possible

Possible investigations

LIKELY: none.

POSSIBLE: urinalysis, FBC, ESR/CRP, rheumatoid factor, uric acid, X-ray.

SMALL PRINT: bone scan, angiography.

NOTE: if the cause is oedema, this will need investigating in its own right (see Swollen ankles, p. 312).

- Urinalysis may reveal glycosuria in previously undiagnosed diabetic with neuropathy (suspicion of neuropathy may in itself require further investigations).
- FBC/ESR/CRP: raised WCC and ESR/CRP in infection and severe inflammation.
- Rheumatoid factor: of prognostic help if foot pain is part of clinical diagnosis of rheumatoid arthritis.
- Uric acid: if gout suspected, especially with recurrent attacks and if considering prophylaxis.
- X-ray useful if suspect possible arthritis, osteomyelitis, march fracture, osteochondritis, radio-opaque foreign body. If clinical suspicion high and X-ray unhelpful, bone scan may be more useful.
- Angiography: if ischaemic foot with rest pain.

TOP TIPS

- The vast majority of causes are obvious from the history or from a cursory examination. The harder you have to think, the more likely that there may be an obscure cause requiring investigation.
- It can be difficult to distinguish gout from a severely inflamed bunion. With gout, the patient may have had previous episodes, the onset tends to be sudden, the joint is extremely tender and joint movements are very limited.
- Important pointers can be picked up in the history, especially for some of the less common causes. Thus, Morton's neuroma causes a sharp pain often radiating to the third and fourth toes, relieved by removing the shoe; plantar fasciitis is described as 'walking on a pebble', especially after resting; and a march fracture results in a pain which initially comes on predictably with exercise and which then becomes continuous, with local bony tenderness and possibly a lump.

- If a known arteriopath complains of pain in the ball of the foot disturbing sleep then the diagnosis is probably critical ischaemia. Refer urgently.
- Fever and systemic illness with localised extreme bone pain and signs of local infection is acute osteomyelitis or septic arthritis until proved otherwise. Admit.
- Pain with no obvious signs – particularly tenderness – in the foot suggests ischaemia, neuropathy or an L5/S1 nerve root lesion.
- If no cause is evident but the patient has very localised sole tenderness away from the heel, consider a foreign body.

NOTES:

HAND AND WRIST PAIN

The GP overview

This may be the presenting problem but just as often it is a 'while I'm here' symptom. The differential diagnosis is quite wide but 'arthritis' is often uppermost in the patient's mind. A brief history and focused examination should provide the correct diagnosis quite rapidly in most cases.

Differential diagnosis

COMMON
- osteoarthritis (especially the carpometacarpal joint of the thumb and the distal interphalangeal joints of the fingers)
- carpal tunnel syndrome
- trauma (e.g. sprain, scaphoid fracture)
- rheumatoid (or other inflammatory) arthritis
- tenosynovitis

OCCASIONAL
- ganglion
- gout
- Raynaud's disease or syndrome
- infection (e.g. paronychia, pulp space)
- work-related upper limb disorder (WRULD)
- trigger thumb or finger
- other nerve entrapment, e.g. ulnar nerve, cervical root pain
- complex regional pain syndrome

RARE
- infected eczema (common, but rarely presents with pain)
- writer's cramp
- peripheral neuropathy
- Dupuytren's contracture (usually painless)
- diabetic arthropathy
- osteomyelitis
- Kienböck's disease (avascular necrosis of the lunate)

Ready reckoner

	OA	Carpal tunnel	Trauma	RA	Tenosynovitis
Symmetrical joint swelling	No	No	No	Yes	No
Abrupt onset	Possible	No	Yes	No	Possible
Paraesthesiae	No	Yes	No	No	No
Worse at night	No	Possible	No	Possible	No
Tendon tender	No	No	Possible	No	Yes

Possible investigations

LIKELY: none.

POSSIBLE: X-ray, FBC, ESR/CRP, rheumatoid factor, uric acid.

SMALL PRINT: blood screen for underlying causes in peripheral neuropathy or Raynaud's syndrome, if clinically indicated.

- ☑ X-ray: may show a fracture in trauma, joint erosions in RA, the typical features of OA, and sclerosis or collapse of the lunate in Kienböck's disease.
- ☑ FBC: Hb may be reduced in inflammatory arthritis; WCC raised in infection.
- ☑ ESR/CRP: raised in infective and inflammatory conditions.
- ☑ Rheumatoid factor: may support a clinical diagnosis of RA.
- ☑ Uric acid: an elevated level (post episode) supports a diagnosis of gout.

TOP TIPS

- ☑ OA of the fingers can be relatively abrupt in onset and inflammatory in appearance compared with OA at other sites.
- ☑ Explore the patient's occupation – this will provide valuable information regarding the possible cause and effect of the problem.
- ☑ Simply asking the patient to point to the site of the pain can help distinguish two of the most commonly confused differentials: OA of the carpometacarpal joint of the thumb and de Quervain's tenosynovitis. In the former the pain is relatively localised to the base of the thumb; in the latter the discomfort – and certainly the tenderness – is more diffuse.
- ☑ Pain from a ganglion can precede the appearance of the ganglion itself – or the ganglion may be fairly subtle, only appearing on wrist flexion.

- Remember that RA is a clinical diagnosis – don't rely on blood tests. Early referral minimises the risk of long-term joint damage.
- If in doubt over tenderness in the anatomical snuff box after a fall on the outstretched hand, refer for A&E assessment – a missed scaphoid fracture can cause long-term problems.
- Do not underestimate pulp space infection – this can cause serious complications such as osteomyelitis or bacterial tenosynovitis. It may need IV antibiotics or incision and drainage.
- Thenar wasting suggests significant compression in carpal tunnel syndrome – refer.

NOTES:

LEG ULCERS

The GP overview

Chronic leg ulcer is a major problem in the UK, costing the National Health Service up to £600m per annum. It is reckoned that nearly 1% of the population may be affected by leg ulceration at some time during their lives. Recurrence is common. The vast majority have a vascular underlying cause.

Differential diagnosis

COMMON
- venous disease: 70–80% of leg ulcers
- peripheral arterial disease: about 15% of leg ulcers
- associated with systemic disease – diabetes (5% of ulcer patients), rheumatoid arthritis (8%), vasculitis
- gross oedema due to systemic causes, e.g. CCF, renal disease, osteoarthritis, severe obesity, prolonged immobility from any cause
- chronic infection, e.g. after trauma, insect bite

OCCASIONAL
- drug misuse
- after primary herpes zoster
- primary malignancy – squamous cell carcinoma, melanoma, malignant change in an existing ulcer
- secondary malignancy – metastases

RARE
- tropical infections
- AIDS
- tuberculosis
- systemic drug reaction
- factitious – self-inflicted (Munchausen's, personality disorder)

Ready reckoner

NOTE: In practice it is very difficult indeed to separate the causes of leg ulcers through clinical examination alone. This is a guide to likely causes only.

	Venous disease	Arterial disease	Systemic disease	Oedema	Infection
Venous eczema/ lipodermatosclerosis	Yes	No	Possible	Possible	No
Weak or absent peripheral pulses	No	Yes	Possible	Possible	No
Generalised illness	No	No	Yes	Possible	Possible
Reduced mobility	Possible	Possible	Possible	Yes	No
Identifiable trigger event	No	No	No	Possible	Possible

Possible investigations

LIKELY: FBC, ESR/CRP, TSH, LFTs, U&E, fasting glucose or HbA1c and RA factor, ABPI.

POSSIBLE: swabs for bacteriology, cardiovascular assessment if appropriate.

SMALL PRINT: Duplex ultrasound.

- FBC, ESR/CRP, CRP, TSH, LFTs, U&E, fasting glucose or HbA1c and RA factor as a basic screen for systemic causes and background disease.
- Swabs for bacteriology are only useful if there is clinical evidence of viable tissue infection, e.g. cellulitis.
- Full cardiovascular assessment if any suspicion of arterial insufficiency.
- Ankle brachial pressure index (ABPI) in both legs by handheld Doppler. Sensitivity of up to 95%; if less than 0.8 assume arterial disease is present. Limited usefulness in patients with microvascular disease, e.g. RA, DM, systemic vasculitis; may cause spuriously high ABPI.
- Specialist: Duplex ultrasound is the investigation of choice to assess arterial and venous insufficiency.

TOP TIPS

- Be systematic in the clinical notes: describe the edge (e.g. rolled, punched-out), base (e.g. sloughy, necrotic, granulating), location, morphology (may help detect rarer causes), and surface area (serial measurements of surface area of an ulcer are a good index of healing).
- Palpation of peripheral pulses is not a reliable guide to arterial sufficiency. Use the ABPI.
- Lipodermatosclerosis is a red or brown patch of skin on the lower leg, usually on the medial side, just above the ankle. This and venous eczema are indications of superficial venous valve failure, even in the absence of varicose veins. They may represent disease amenable to surgery, so refer for a vascular opinion.

- Deep ulcers involving deep fascia, tendon, periosteum or bone may well have an arterial component.
- Mixed ulcer aetiology may confuse the clinical picture and make treatment choices harder. Refer for a specialist opinion if in any doubt.
- More than 50% of leg ulcer patients are sensitive to one or more allergens, including lanolin, topical antibiotics, cetyl stearyl alcohols, balsam of Peru and parabens. These may contribute to non-healing and cause discomfort to the patient. Refer the patient for patch testing if dermatitis is associated with a leg ulcer.
- Topical antibiotics do not contribute to healing and are frequent sensitisers – avoid using them.

- Pain from an ulcer is most frequently associated with an arterial aetiology.
- Refer for biopsy if the ulcer has an atypical appearance or distribution, or fails to heal within 12 weeks of treatment. Beware neoplastic change in an existing ulcer. This is rare, but not to be missed.
- Compression bandaging is dangerous in diabetes and arterial insufficiency. Do not prescribe it until they are ruled out. If in doubt about ABPI, refer for a vascular opinion.

NOTES:

MULTIPLE JOINT PAIN

The GP overview

The range of causes of multiple joint pain spans acute, chronic and chronic relapsing conditions. In the elderly, the commonest problem is multiple osteoarthritis; in middle age, inflammatory conditions predominate; and in the young, systemic conditions are more likely.

Differential diagnosis

COMMON
- rheumatoid arthritis (RA)
- psoriatic arthropathy
- viral polyarthritis, e.g. hepatitis, rubella
- connective tissue diseases, e.g. SLE, systemic sclerosis, polymyositis, polyarteritis nodosa, giant cell arteritis
- multiple osteoarthritis (OA)

OCCASIONAL
- the spondoarthritides: ankylosing spondylitis, Reiter's disease, enteropathic arthritis, Behçet's syndrome, juvenile chronic arthritis
- Henoch–Schönlein syndrome
- malignancy (usually secondary)
- iatrogenic: corticosteroid therapy, isoniazid, hydralazine
- hypertrophic pulmonary osteoarthropathy (due to lung cancer)
- sarcoidosis

RARE
- sickle-cell crisis
- amyloidosis
- rheumatic fever
- atypical systemic infections, e.g. Lyme disease, Weil's disease, brucellosis, syphilis (secondary)
- decompression sickness (the bends)

Ready reckoner

	RA	Psoriasis	Viral	Connective tissue	OA
Symmetrical	Yes	Possible	Possible	Possible	Possible
Rash	No	Yes	Possible	Possible	No
Fever, malaise	Possible	No	Yes	Possible	No
Young patient	Possible	Possible	Possible	Possible	No
Self-limiting	No	No	Yes	No	No

Possible investigations

LIKELY: FBC, ESR/CRP, autoantibodies.

POSSIBLE: urinalysis, U&E, HLA-B27, joint X-rays, synovial fluid aspiration.

SMALL PRINT: blood film, serology, creatine phosphokinase, CXR, bone scan, Kveim test.

- FBC, ESR/CRP, blood film: WCC and ESR/CRP raised in acute inflammation and infection. Anaemia of chronic disease may be seen, and blood film will reveal sickle cell.
- Autoantibodies: rheumatoid factor is positive in most cases of RA, but is also positive in many autoimmune diseases and chronic infections; antinuclear factor is positive in 90% of cases of SLE but a similar result is obtained in 30% of cases of RA and also in many other diseases.
- Urinalysis: may reveal proteinuria or haematuria if there is renal involvement in connective tissue disease.
- U&E: to check for renal failure via renal involvement in multisystem connective tissue disease.
- HLA-B27: a high prevalence in spondoarthritides.
- Serology: may be useful to diagnose viral, or atypical systemic, infections. ASO titres, if rising, suggest recent streptococcal infection (e.g. in rheumatic fever).
- Creatine phosphokinase: elevated in polymyositis.
- Joint X-rays: hand X-rays may show characteristic features helping to distinguish between RA and psoriatic arthritis; pelvic and lumbar spine X-rays may show the typical changes of ankylosing spondylitis (if negative, and clinical suspicion high, a bone scan may be helpful); X-rays of affected joints may confirm clinical diagnosis of OA.
- CXR: may reveal lung malignancy.
- Synovial fluid analysis: helps distinguish inflammatory from infective and crystal arthropathies.
- Sarcoidosis: Kveim test may help confirm diagnosis.

TOP TIPS

- ▧ The connective tissue diseases can all affect almost every organ system. Take a full history so as not to miss a clue or complication.
- ▧ Check the skin as this may contribute to the diagnosis (e.g. scaly rash in psoriasis, butterfly rash in SLE, thickening of skin in sclerosis and heliotrope rash in dermatomyositis).
- ▧ Don't overvalue autoimmune blood tests. Most diagnoses of arthritis are clinical, blood tests simply providing confirmatory or prognostic information.

- ▧ Suspect Reiter's syndrome in a young male with an inflammatory oligoarthritis of the lower limbs.
- ▧ An insidious onset of symmetrical polyarthritis in the 30–50 age range, with early morning stiffness, pain and swelling of hands and feet, suggests RA.
- ▧ Pain in the wrists and ankles of a middle-aged or elderly smoker with clubbing and chest symptoms strongly suggests hypertrophic pulmonary osteoarthropathy caused by underlying lung cancer.
- ▧ Don't overlook the patient's occupation as this may be relevant in certain cases: for example, in vets and farm workers, brucellosis and Weil's disease are possible infective causes.

NOTES:

PAINFUL MUSCLES

The GP overview

This symptom has a multitude of causes. A careful history is required to distinguish between muscle and joint pain, and between muscle pain and weakness. In some of the underlying pathologies, these symptoms may coexist. Cramp, causing very transient muscle pain, is covered elsewhere (see Calf pain, p. 288).

Differential diagnosis

COMMON
- overuse (including strain injury)
- acute viral illness
- depression
- polymyalgia rheumatica (PMR)
- side effects of statins (myalgia much more common than myositis)

OCCASIONAL
- vitamin D deficiency
- referred joint pain (e.g. from hip to thigh, neck to shoulder, shoulder to arm)
- fibromyalgia
- chronic fatigue syndrome
- connective tissue disease, e.g. RA, SLE, polyarteritis nodosa (PAN), scleroderma
- peripheral vascular disease: intermittent claudication
- neuropathy: diabetic, alcoholic
- Bornholm disease (epidemic myalgia, devil's grip)
- hypothyroidism
- drugs: statins, clofibrate, street drug withdrawal, chemotherapy, lithium, cimetidine

RARE
- polymyositis (usually more weakness than pain)
- adult and childhood dermatomyositis
- underlying malignancy
- porphyria
- Guillain–Barré syndrome and poliomyelitis

Ready reckoner

	Overuse	Viral illness	Depression	PMR	Statin side effect
Sudden onset	Yes	Yes	No	Possible	Possible
Morning stiffness	Yes	Possible	No	Yes	No
Vague generalised	No	Possible	Yes	No	Possible
Persistent	No	No	Yes	Yes	Yes
Muscle tenderness	Yes	Possible	No	Possible	Possible

Possible investigations

LIKELY: FBC, ESR/CRP.

POSSIBLE: urinalysis, autoimmune blood tests, TFT, LFT, blood sugar or HbA1c, creatine phosphokinase (CPK), vitamin D levels.

SMALL PRINT: joint and chest X-rays; in secondary care, angiography, electromyography, muscle biopsy, lumbar puncture, urinary porphyrins.

- Urinalysis: glycosuria in undiagnosed diabetes.
- FBC and ESR/CRP: Hb may be depressed in connective tissue disease and PMR. WCC and ESR/CRP raised in any inflammatory disorder (ESR more useful than CRP in PMR); MCV elevated in hypothyroidism and alcohol abuse.
- Autoimmune blood tests: may be helpful if connective tissue disorder suspected.
- TFT: will confirm hypothyroidism.
- Blood sugar or HbA1c, LFT: the former to confirm diabetes; the latter may help in confirming an alcohol problem. Both may cause a neuropathy resulting in muscle pain.
- CPK: raised in acute inflammatory and viral myopathies.
- Vitamin D levels: vitamin D deficiency is increasingly being recognised and may present with muscle pain and/or weakness.
- Joint X-rays: if referred pain from primary joint pathology suspected.
- Angiography: for peripheral vascular disease.
- Electromyography and muscle biopsy (both in secondary care): to confirm diagnosis of polymyositis or dermatomyositis.
- Lumbar puncture: to examine CSF in hospital in suspected Guillain–Barré syndrome or poliomyelitis.
- Urinary porphyrins: to exclude porphyria.
- Other investigations for suspected underlying malignancy, e.g. CXR.

TOP TIPS

- ⬜ In polysymptomatic patients with muscle pain but no objective signs and normal blood tests, consider fibromyalgia, depression and chronic fatigue (*Note:* these problems may coexist).
- ⬜ The diagnosis of PMR is clinched by a trial of prednisolone (20 mg/day). In PMR, this treatment should lead to total resolution of symptoms within a few days.
- ⬜ Muscle pain is more likely to be associated with significant pathology in the very young and old than the middle-aged, when psychological causes and overuse are the most likely.

- ⬜ Always remember PMR in the older patient complaining of aching pain and stiffness in the hip and shoulder girdle muscles which is worse in the mornings.
- ⬜ If considering PMR, or initiating treatment in this condition, enquire after symptoms of temporal arteritis. About 30% of patients develop this complication, and are at risk of blindness.
- ⬜ Muscle pain with significant and progressive weakness (e.g. difficulty climbing stairs or getting out of a chair) suggests polymyositis, hypothyroidism, vitamin D deficiency or malignancy.
- ⬜ Significant underlying disease (e.g. PMR, polymyositis, dermatomyositis or connective tissue disease) is likely if there is an arthritis associated with the muscle pain.

NOTES:

RECURRENT HIP AREA PAIN IN AN ADULT

The GP overview

Hip area pain is a common presentation in the middle-aged and elderly, and the patient will often attribute it to osteoarthritis. This diagnosis may well be correct, although the differential is wide – besides, the patient's view of what actually constitutes the 'hip' may be at odds with the anatomical truth. The differential for the child with hip pain is very different – see Limp in a child, p. 209.

Differential diagnosis

COMMON
- muscular/ligamentous strain
- osteoarthritis
- trochanteric bursitis
- referred from back
- meralgia paraesthetica

OCCASIONAL
- inflammatory arthritis
- avascular necrosis
- hernia
- complications of a total hip replacement, e.g. loosening, infection
- spinal stenosis
- iliotibial band syndrome
- acetabular labral tear

RARE
- impacted fracture
- dislocation
- bony pathology, e.g. secondaries, Paget's

Ready reckoner

	Muscular/ ligament	Osteoarthritis	Trochanteric bursitis	Referred from back	Meralgia paraesthetica
Pain lying on affected side	Possible	No	Yes	No	No
Leg numbness	No	No	No	Possible	Yes
Painful hip movement	Yes	Yes	Possible	No	No
Pain mainly in groin	Possible	Yes	No	Possible	No
Coexisting back pain	No	Possible	No	Yes	No

Possible investigations

LIKELY: X-ray.

POSSIBLE: FBC, CRP, autoantibodies, HLA-B27, alkaline phosphatase, urinalysis.

SMALL PRINT: arthroscopy, bone scan, lumbar spine MRI (all in hospital).

- X-ray: may show evidence of osteoarthritis, avascular necrosis, fracture, dislocation, hip replacement loosening and bony pathology. Spinal X-ray may reveal spinal pathology as a cause.
- FBC, CRP: CRP may be elevated and Hb reduced in inflammatory arthritis. CRP and WCC raised in infection of joint prosthesis.
- Autoantibodies: for clues about the aetiology of inflammatory arthritis.
- HLA-B27: a high prevalence in spondoarthrities.
- Alkaline phosphatase: raised in Paget's disease.
- Urinalysis: may reveal proteinuria or haematuria if there is renal involvement in inflammatory arthritis.
- Arthroscopy: diagnostic and potentially therapeutic in labral tear.
- Bone scan: may reveal bony secondaries.
- Lumbar spine MRI: for evidence of spinal stenosis; might reveal other causes of pain referred from spine.

TOP TIPS

- Check what the patient means by 'hip'. Most don't realise that the hip joint is actually in the groin.
- An X-ray may not be necessary, even if the clinical picture suggests hip arthritis – but the patient may well expect one, so ensure it is at least discussed.
- Examine the patient standing up – this may reveal a hernia as the cause.
- Localised lateral pain aggravated by lying on the affected side is likely to be caused by trochanteric bursitis.

- ◪ Remember the possibility of loosening or infection in joint replacements.
- ◪ Consider avascular necrosis if a patient on long-term steroids develops severe hip pain.
- ◪ Beware that the elderly can sometimes remain weight bearing – albeit with pain and a limp – after an impacted hip fracture.
- ◪ Significant depression may aggravate or result from hip arthritis pain – consider a trial of antidepressants.

NOTES:

RECURRENT KNEE PAIN

The GP overview

Recurrent knee pain is a very common presentation with a wide differential. Classification of causes isn't helped by changing and confusing nomenclature. As ever in general practice, a careful history and examination will provide useful clues – but management will often be dictated more by degree of disability and the patient's wishes than by making a precise diagnosis.

Differential diagnosis

COMMON
- ligament sprain/minor soft tissue injury
- osteoarthritis
- cartilage injury
- chondromalacia patellae/patellofemoral pain
- Osgood–Schlatter's disease

OCCASIONAL
- recurrent monoarthritis, e.g. gout, pseudogout, Reiter's
- as part of polyarthritis, e.g. rheumatoid, ankylosing spondylitis, psoriatic arthritis
- iliotibial tract syndrome
- bursitis
- referred from hip or back
- ligament rupture
- patellar tendonitis
- Baker's cyst
- loose body
- bone disease, e.g. Paget's
- recurrent dislocation of the patella
- medial shelf syndrome
- osteochondritis dissecans

RARE
- haemochromatosis
- recurrent haemarthroses, e.g. coagulation disorder
- osteosarcoma

Ready reckoner

	Ligament sprain/ soft tissue	Osteoarthritis	Cartilage injury	Chondromalacia patellae/ patellofemoral pain	Osgood– Schlatter's
Effusion	No	Possible	Possible	Possible	No
Specific injury	Yes	No	Yes	No	No
Locking	No	Possible	Possible	No	No
Both knees affected	No	Possible	No	Possible	Possible
More common in women	No	No	No	Yes	No

Possible investigations

LIKELY: X-ray.

POSSIBLE: FBC, CRP, uric acid, MRI, autoantibodies.

SMALL PRINT: HLA-B27, joint aspiration, hip or back investigations if referred pain suspected, alkaline phosphatase, serum ferritin, coagulation screen.

- X-ray: may give clues to many of the possible causes, or confirmatory evidence when clinical suspicion is high – for example, with osteoarthritis, bony loose body, Paget's, osteochondritis dissecans.
- FBC, CRP: CRP elevated and Hb may be reduced in inflammatory polyarthritis.
- Uric acid: typically elevated in gout.
- MRI: useful to assess soft tissue such as cartilage, especially if surgery is being considered.
- Autoantibodies: if inflammatory polyarthritis suspected.
- HLA-B27: a high prevalence in spondoarthritides.
- Joint aspiration: may be diagnostically useful if an effusion is present – for example, revealing positively birefringent crystals in pseudogout. In practice, usually performed after specialist referral.
- Hip or back investigations: appropriate radiology may be necessary if it is thought the knee pain is referred from these areas.
- Alkaline phosphatase: elevated in Paget's.
- Serum ferritin: elevated in haemochromatosis.
- Coagulation screen: if coagulopathy suspected.

TOP TIPS

- Patients place great value on X-rays whereas, in practice, they may contribute little to management of straightforward recurrent knee pain. To prevent an unsatisfactory outcome, consider proactively broaching the fact that an X-ray may be unnecessary.

- Insisting that the patient accurately localises the pain – if possible – may usefully limit the diagnostic possibilities.
- 'Straightforward' osteoarthritis can become quite suddenly more painful, often for no obvious reason – exacerbations and remissions are part of the natural history of the disease.
- Keen sports people often present with recurrent knee pain and are unlikely to indulge in the GP's time-honoured 'wait and see' approach. Earlier investigation or intervention may prove necessary.

Red flags

- Do not forget that knee pain may be referred – if the cause isn't immediately apparent, examine the hip, especially in children.
- Anterior cruciate ligament injury is quite easily missed in casualty in the acute stage. It may only present later with an unstable knee.
- Osteosarcomas are rare – but most commonly occur near the knee. Beware of unexplained constant, increasing pain waking the patient at night. Swelling and inflammation will only appear later.

NOTES:

SWOLLEN ANKLES

The GP overview

This is one of the commonest presenting complaints in the elderly and, in this age group, may be linked to recurrent falls. As a result, it is frequently the reason for a home visit request. In younger age groups, it is much rarer, but much more likely to signify serious pathology.

Differential diagnosis

COMMON
- congestive cardiac failure (CCF)
- drug reaction – especially calcium antagonists
- gravitational (venous insufficiency, often with poor mobility)
- obesity
- pelvic mass (including pregnancy)

OCCASIONAL
- cirrhosis
- premenstrual syndrome
- anaemia
- renal: acute or chronic nephritis, nephrotic syndrome
- protein-losing enteropathy, e.g. coeliac disease, inflammatory bowel disease

RARE
- malnutrition
- inferior vena cava thrombosis
- filariasis
- Milroy's disease (hereditary lymphoedema)
- ancylostomiasis (hookworm)
- angioneurotic oedema

Ready reckoner

	CCF	Drug reaction	Gravitational	Obesity	Pelvic mass
Shortness of breath on exertion	Yes	No	No	Possible	Possible
Altered breath sounds	Yes	Possible	No	No	No
Less swollen in the morning	Possible	Possible	Yes	Possible	Possible
Taking oedema-genic drug	Possible	Yes	No	No	No
Other symptoms or signs	Yes	Yes	No	No	Yes

Possible investigations

LIKELY: urinalysis, FBC, U&E, LFT.

POSSIBLE: TFT.

SMALL PRINT: CXR, pelvic ultrasound, further investigation of underlying cause.

- Urinalysis: for proteinuria.
- FBC: look for anaemia of chronic disorder, raised MCV (alcohol abuse).
- U&E: will reveal underlying renal failure; sodium low in CCF and cirrhosis.
- LFT: may reveal hypoproteinaemia (e.g. in cirrhosis, protein-losing enteropathy and nephrotic syndrome).
- CXR: pulmonary oedema and pleural effusion in CCF.
- Pelvic ultrasound: for pelvic mass.
- Further investigation of underlying cause: this might involve ECG, BNP and echocardiography (CCF), CT scan (pelvic mass), renal biopsy (nephritis) and bowel investigations (enteropathy).

TOP TIPS

- In the elderly, the cause is often multifactorial, with immobility playing a major role.
- Proper assessment can take time: consider spreading the work over a couple of consultations, using the intervening time to arrange and assess investigations.
- Ankle swelling is usually symmetrical, though venous insufficiency in particular can affect one side much more than the other. But if only one ankle is swollen, consider deep vein thrombosis, a ruptured Baker's cyst or cellulitis.
- Don't forget that many drugs (such as calcium antagonists and NSAIDs) can cause marked ankle swelling.

- If no cause is obvious in an elderly person, examine the abdomen and also consider a rectal examination.
- The younger the patient, the greater the chance of significant pathology – especially renal.
- Marked swelling of recent and sudden onset is likely to be significant regardless of age.

NOTES:

SWOLLEN CALF

The GP overview

Such has been the publicity about 'economy class syndrome' that this presentation – and the closely related symptom, 'calf pain' (see p. 288) – has become quite common. The worry the patient has about a possible DVT can prove quite 'infectious', with the GP anxious not to miss this significant problem. In most cases, a careful history, backed up by appropriate examination, should reveal the true cause.

Differential diagnosis

COMMON

- cellulitis
- most causes of swollen ankles (see p. 312)
- muscle strain/rupture (especially rupture of plantaris tendon)
- ruptured Baker's cyst
- DVT

OCCASIONAL

- ruptured Achilles tendon
- varicose eczema
- phlebitis

RARE

- muscle herniation through fascia (especially tibialis anterior)
- muscular neoplasm
- pseudohypertrophy (as in muscular dystrophy)

Ready reckoner

	Cellulitis	Swollen ankles	Muscular	Baker's cyst	DVT
Fever	Yes	No	No	No	Possible
Bilateral	Possible	Possible	No	No	Possible
Sudden pain	No	No	Yes	Possible	Possible
Previous swelling behind knee	No	No	No	Yes	No
Skin red	Yes	Possible	No	No	Possible

Possible investigations

LIKELY: none (unless sent to hospital).

POSSIBLE: FBC, ESR/CRP and other investigations for swollen ankles (see p. 312); usually in hospital – D-dimer, ultrasound, venography.

SMALL PRINT: (in hospital) radio-iodine labelled fibrinogen uptake test.

- FBC, ESR/CRP: elevated white cell count and ESR/CRP in cellulitis.
- D-dimer: raised level suggests DVT but is not conclusive.
- Ultrasound: may help diagnose DVT and useful in confirming ruptured Baker's cyst as the cause.
- Venography, radio-iodine labelled fibrinogen uptake test: hospital test which may be used to confirm DVT.

TOP TIPS

- The swelling resulting from a muscle rupture can be impressive – but a typical history with pain (described as 'Like being shot in the calf') preceding the swelling should clinch the correct diagnosis.
- Varicose eczema is often misdiagnosed as cellulitis. Clues are that it is commonly bilateral, itches more than hurts and is not accompanied by fever.
- Anxiety about possible DVT may cloud the presentation: careful questioning may reveal that swelling is, in fact, long-standing and/or bilateral, making DVT very unlikely.

☑ Patients with unexplained DVT are three to four times more likely than controls to have an underlying malignancy – so, once the DVT has been dealt with, consider appropriate investigation.

☑ In high-risk patients – such as those who have just returned from a long haul flight – your index of suspicion for DVT should be raised.

☑ When the history suggests muscular rupture, ensure that the Achilles tendon is intact.

NOTES:

NECK

Difficulty swallowing

Hoarseness

Neck lumps

Sore throat

Stiff neck

Stridor in children

DIFFICULTY SWALLOWING

The GP overview

This symptom can mean several things, and a careful history is necessary to tease out the precise problem: difficulty in initiating swallowing; a sensation of food sticking somewhere; painful swallowing; also included here is the sensation of 'something in the throat' even when not trying to swallow anything.

Differential diagnosis

COMMON
- globus hystericus
- any painful pharyngeal condition, e.g. pharyngitis
- GORD
- benign stricture
- oesophageal carcinoma

OCCASIONAL
- pharyngeal pouch
- pharyngeal carcinoma
- compression by mediastinal tumours (e.g. lymphoma, bronchial carcinoma)
- oesophageal achalasia
- gastric carcinoma
- xerostomia (the elderly, post-parotidectomy and Sjögren's syndrome)
- foreign body
- drugs: NSAID-associated oesophagitis, failure to take bisphosphonate tablets correctly

RARE
- Plummer–Vinson syndrome
- Chagas's disease (South American trypanosomal infection)
- scleroderma (CREST syndrome), polymyositis and dermatomyositis
- neurological disorders, e.g. myasthenia gravis, bulbar palsy
- motor neurone disease

Ready reckoner

	Globus	GORD	Stricture	Oesophageal carcinoma	Painful pharynx
Weight loss	No	No	Possible	Yes	No
Intermittent	Yes	Yes	No	No	No
Progressive	No	No	Yes	Yes	No
Reflux of unchanged food	No	No	Possible	Yes	No
Retrosternal pain	No	Yes	Possible	Possible	No

Possible investigations

LIKELY: (unless obvious globus or local pharyngeal cause) FBC, ESR/CRP, barium swallow or endoscopy.

POSSIBLE: CXR, LFT.

SMALL PRINT: pharyngeal swab, CT scan thorax.

- ☑ FBC and ESR/CRP: may reveal evidence of malignancy or iron-deficiency anaemia.
- ☑ LFT if malignancy suspected: abnormality suggests hepatic spread.
- ☑ Barium swallow useful in the frail and to safely demonstrate stricture or motility problems if no absolute dysphagia for liquids (risk of aspiration).
- ☑ Flexible upper GI endoscopy allows visualisation and biopsy of suspicious lesions.
- ☑ Throat swab occasionally helpful in painful pharyngeal lesions.
- ☑ CXR if suspicion of mediastinal tumour of any cause.
- ☑ CT scan or further imaging may be arranged by the specialist to further define mediastinal tumours.

TOP TIPS

- ☑ A young patient under stress who can swallow food and drink without problems but who feels there is 'something stuck' almost certainly has globus. Reassurance usually resolves the situation.
- ☑ Remember to ask about medication – recent onset of painful dysphagia may be caused by severe oesophagitis secondary to drugs such as alendronate, NSAIDs and slow-release potassium supplements.
- ☑ Take time with the history: difficulty in swallowing can mean a number of different things, and the diagnosis is much more likely to be revealed by careful questioning than by examination.

- Recent onset of progressive dysphagia with weight loss in an elderly patient is caused by oesophageal carcinoma until proved otherwise.
- A palpable hard lymph node in the left supraclavicular fossa (Troisier's sign) is strongly associated with gastric carcinoma.
- Beware of patients who have a long history of oesophagitis but who complain of increasing or unusual dysphagia: they may have developed a stricture, or even a carcinoma.
- If endoscopy does not reveal a cause but the symptom continues, remember rarer causes, such as extrinsic compression on the oesophagus or a neurological problem. Consider a barium swallow, or referral to a neurologist if there are other neurological symptoms or signs.

NOTES:

HOARSENESS

The GP overview

Hoarseness may start suddenly and last a few days (acute), or arise gradually and continue for weeks or months (chronic). The history will clarify this and point the way forward in management. Acute hoarseness rarely causes any diagnostic problem or concern; the less common chronic case raises more worrying possibilities and usually requires referral.

Differential diagnosis

COMMON
- acute viral laryngitis
- voice overuse (shouting, screaming)
- hypothyroidism
- smoking
- sinusitis

OCCASIONAL
- GORD
- benign tumours: singer's nodes, polyps
- crico-arytenoid rheumatoid arthritis
- functional (hysterical) aphonia

RARE
- acute epiglottitis
- laryngeal carcinoma
- recurrent laryngeal nerve palsy
- physical trauma (e.g. after intubation)
- chemical inhalation trauma
- rare inflammatory lesions (e.g. TB, syphilis)

Ready reckoner

	Acute laryngitis	Overuse	Hypothyroidism	Smoking	Sinusitis
Recent illness	Yes	No	Possible	No	Yes
Tired, cold and slowed up	No	No	Yes	No	No
Fever and malaise	Possible	No	No	No	Yes
Symptoms chronic	No	Possible	Yes	Yes	No
Facial pain and catarrh	No	No	No	No	Yes

Possible investigations

LIKELY: none.

POSSIBLE: TFT, CXR, direct or indirect laryngoscopy.

SMALL PRINT: throat swab.

- TFT: in chronic hoarseness to exclude hypothyroidism.
- CXR: to check for thoracic lesions causing recurrent laryngeal nerve palsy.
- Indirect laryngoscopy: useful for a GP with the necessary skills; most will refer to an ENT specialist.
- Direct laryngoscopy: using a flexible fibre-optic endoscope. This is a specialist investigation allowing close-up views and biopsy of suspicious lesions.
- Throat swab: useful, very rarely, if hoarseness is associated with a persisting pharyngitis.

TOP TIPS

- In acute laryngitis, don't forget to tell the patient to rest the voice, and remember that occupational factors are important: use of voice (e.g. by telephonists) or working in smoky environment (e.g. a pub) will aggravate and prolong symptoms, causing diagnostic confusion.
- If you suspect a malignancy, arrange an urgent CXR immediately prior to referral. The referral can then be made to the correct specialist (chest rather than ENT) if a lung lesion is present, thus expediting appropriate management.
- Don't forget transient hoarseness caused by intubation – GPs are seeing this increasingly often as patients spend less post-operative time in hospital.

- Every adult patient with hoarseness for 3 weeks or more showing no signs of improvement has carcinoma of the larynx until proved otherwise.
- GORD is a common cause in the elderly, but beware of making this diagnosis without specialist investigation first.
- Epiglottitis is rare but if you suspect it in any patient, admit immediately – and don't examine the throat.
- Hypothyroidism is easily overlooked – prompt diagnosis can save unnecessary anxiety and investigation.

NOTES:

NECK LUMPS

The GP overview

A lump in the neck usually means just one thing to a patient: cancer. This is rarely the cause in practice, and a careful examination and explanation can be more anxiolytic than a bucket-load of benzodiazepines. Occasionally further investigation is needed.

Differential diagnosis

COMMON
- ☑ reactive lymphadenitis due to a local infection
- ☑ prominent normal lymph nodes
- ☑ goitre
- ☑ sebaceous cyst
- ☑ thyroglossal cyst

OCCASIONAL
- ☑ branchial cyst
- ☑ pharyngeal pouch
- ☑ cervical rib
- ☑ actinomycosis
- ☑ primary lymphoma or secondary neoplastic metastasis

RARE
- ☑ tuberculosis of cervical lymph nodes (king's evil; scrofula)
- ☑ thyroid carcinoma
- ☑ carotid body tumour or aneurysm
- ☑ sarcoidosis
- ☑ cystic hygroma

Ready reckoner

	Lymphadenitis	Normal nodes	Goitre	Sebaceous cyst	Thyroglossal cyst
Tender	Yes	No	Possible	No	No
Other symptoms	Yes	No	Possible	No	No
Moves with swallowing	No	No	Yes	No	Yes
Midline	No	No	No	No	Yes
Fixed to skin	No	No	No	Yes	No

Possible investigations

LIKELY: TFTs if thyroid swelling.

POSSIBLE: FBC, ESR, CXR.

SMALL PRINT: thyroid ultrasound, radioisotope studies, barium swallow, biopsy.

- TFT in all cases of thyroid enlargement: may reveal hypo- or hyperthyroidism.
- FBC and ESR in persistent enlarged nodes: check WCC and investigate further if abnormal or if ESR high.
- CXR: may reveal primary lung carcinoma, lymphoma, or other more obscure pathologies.
- Thyroid ultrasound and/or radioiodine studies if lump felt within the thyroid – usually arranged by endocrinologist after referral.
- Barium swallow: to confirm and outline a pharyngeal pouch.
- Biopsy: specialist procedure to establish nature of a persistent, suspicious neck lump.

TOP TIPS

- Establish the patient's concerns: cancer fear is common with this symptom.
- Unless the lump is obviously suspicious, employ the 'diagnostic use of time' – a judicious delay often resolves the problem, or it may reveal the true diagnosis.
- Suspicious lymphadenopathy usually involves a single, gradually enlarging and non-tender lymph node.
- Children with normal or reactive neck glands are often presented by anxious parents. Take time to explain the nature of the problem to properly allay fears and prevent inappropriate repeat attendances.

- A neoplastic-type lymph node enlargement without any obvious cause should be referred urgently for detailed ENT assessment.
- A neck lump fixed to skin and without a punctum should arouse suspicion: urgent biopsy should be done once a primary ENT tumour is ruled out.
- Dysphagia with a neck lump is a serious symptom unless associated with a transient sore throat. Further investigation by endoscopy is necessary.
- Beware of a hard swelling developing rapidly in the thyroid – carcinoma must be excluded.

NOTES:

SORE THROAT

The GP overview

This presenting symptom is the king of superlatives in general practice. It is the commonest – the average GP will see about 120 cases each year – the most over-treated, the most controversial and usually the most mundane. It is also probably the most welcome, as consultations are often short, even when self-management is explained rather than a prescription given.

Differential diagnosis

COMMON
- mild viral pharyngitis (with URTI)
- tonsillitis/streptococcal pharyngitis ('strep throat')
- glandular fever
- quinsy (peritonsillar abscess)
- oropharyngeal candidiasis

OCCASIONAL
- GORD
- glossopharyngeal neuralgia and cervicogenic nerve root pain
- trauma: foreign body or scratch from badly chewed crispy food
- other viral or bacterial infections, e.g. Vincent's angina, herpangina, herpes simplex, gonorrhoea
- aphthous ulceration
- acute or subacute thyroiditis

RARE
- cardiac angina
- carotidynia
- blood dyscrasia (including iatrogenic)
- epiglottitis
- diphtheria
- oropharyngeal carcinoma
- retropharyngeal abscess

Ready reckoner

	Mild viral	'Strep throat'	Glandular fever	Quinsy	Oropharyngeal candidiasis
Cervical lymphadenopathy	Possible	Yes	Yes	Yes	No
Purulent throat	No	Yes	Possible	Possible	No
High fever	No	Yes	Yes	Yes	No
Unilaterally swollen	No	Possible	No	Yes	No
URTI symptoms	Yes	No	No	No	No

Possible investigations

LIKELY: none.

POSSIBLE: throat swab, FBC, Paul–Bunnell test.

SMALL PRINT: upper GI endoscopy, biopsy, cardiac investigation (all secondary care).

- ☑ Throat swab: use is controversial, mainly because of low specificity and sensitivity. Practical use only in persistent sore throat or treatment failure.
- ☑ FBC: may show atypical lymphocytes in glandular fever; also will reveal any underlying blood dyscrasia.
- ☑ Paul–Bunnell test for glandular fever if malaise and fatigue persist.
- ☑ Upper GI endoscopy may be necessary to diagnose GORD.
- ☑ X-ray/laryngoscopy: if suspicion of foreign body.
- ☑ Cardiac investigation: in rare case when referred symptoms cause pain in throat.
- ☑ Biopsy of suspicious lesions important to investigate possible malignancy.

TOP TIPS

- ☑ Consultations for severe sore throats usually boil down to a decision whether or not to prescribe antibiotics. There is no easy or reliable way to distinguish clinically between bacterial and viral causes, so the situation becomes an exercise in pragmatism, though the Centor criteria may help. Even in 'true' streptococcal throats, antibiotic treatment probably only reduces the duration of symptoms by about 24 hours and is unlikely to influence the likelihood of complications.
- ☑ Mild sore throat with an URTI is usually just one of a 'package' of symptoms presented, along with rhinorrhoea, cough, headache and so on. The cause is invariably viral and antibiotics have no role to play.
- ☑ Throat swabs only help management in obscure or persistent cases (and even then usually contribute little).
- ☑ In adolescents and young adults whom you decide to treat with antibiotics for 'strep throat', explain that the symptoms can also be caused by other infections such as glandular fever. This will help maintain the patients' confidence in you if they return with the sore throat persisting after the course of antibiotics.

Red flags

☑ Remember that this apparently trivial symptom can occasionally herald a serious problem. In particular, enquire about medication (the first sign of drug-induced agranulocytosis may be a sore throat).

☑ A true foreign body stuck in the throat will lodge in the supraglottic area and may not be seen orally. Refer if in doubt.

☑ Admit if any suspicion of epiglottitis – and do not examine the throat.

☑ Consider a possible underlying problem (such as diabetes or immunosuppression) in the younger patient with oropharyngeal candidiasis which has no obvious cause.

☑ Quinsy can cause a respiratory obstruction. Never attempt conservative management, but admit for surgical drainage.

☑ Florid 'tonsillitis' is unusual in the middle-aged or elderly – consider investigations for a blood disorder or oropharyngeal carcinoma.

NOTES:

STIFF NECK

The GP overview

The most common causes of acute neck stiffness are benign and easily managed in general practice. However, this symptom causes disproportionate panic in parents of febrile children thanks to extensive media coverage of meningitis. This anxiety can spill over into adult illness behaviour, with the result that a troublesome but harmless symptom may be misinterpreted as the harbinger of serious pathology.

Differential diagnosis

COMMON
- acute torticollis (positional, draughts)
- cervical spondylosis
- viral URTI with cervical lymphadenitis
- whiplash injury
- meningism due to systemic infection (e.g. pneumonia)

OCCASIONAL
- other forms of arthritis, e.g. rheumatoid (RA) and ankylosing spondylitis
- abscess in the neck
- hysteria
- intracerebral haemorrhage
- cerebral tumour (primary or secondary)

RARE
- meningitis
- vertebral fracture
- bone tumour (primary or secondary)
- atypical infections: tetanus, leptospirosis, sandfly fever, psittacosis
- brain abscess

Ready reckoner

	Torticollis	Cervical spondylosis	URTI	Whiplash	Meningism
Other symptoms	No	Possible	Yes	Possible	Yes
Recurrent	No	Yes	No	Possible	No
Enlarged lymph nodes	No	No	Yes	No	Possible
Neck asymmetrical	Yes	Possible	No	Possible	No
Fever	No	No	Yes	No	Yes

Possible investigations

LIKELY: none.

POSSIBLE: FBC, Paul–Bunnell test, ESR/CRP, rheumatoid factor, HLA-B27.

SMALL PRINT: bone biochemistry, X-ray cervical spine, bone scan, other hospital-based tests.

- ▱ FBC and Paul–Bunnell: in unresolved or resistant URTI, check these parameters if glandular fever suspected.
- ▱ ESR/CRP, rheumatoid factor and HLA-B27: will help in the diagnosis of possible RA and ankylosing spondylitis in the young and middle-aged with unresolving neck stiffness.
- ▱ Neck X-ray: for possible fracture (at hospital); of limited value in cervical spondylosis – symptoms do not correlate well with X-ray findings. May reveal serious bone pathology, but bone scan more useful for this.
- ▱ Bone biochemistry: consider this if bony secondaries or myeloma are possible diagnoses.
- ▱ Hospital-based tests: these might include lumbar puncture (for meningitis) and scans for cerebral lesions.

TOP TIPS

- ▱ Neck tenderness due to cervical lymphadenopathy in an URTI is infinitely more common than meningitis, but is often misreported as 'neck stiffness'.
- ▱ Only advise soft collars in the majority of stiff necks for a maximum of 48 hours. Though comfortable, they tend to delay resolution. Instead, suggest adequate analgesia, heat and mobilisation.
- ▱ Warn patients with whiplash injury that symptoms may take many months to settle completely – this saves repeated futile and frustrating consultations.

- Meningococcal petechiae are usually a late sign and can be missed unless the febrile child with a stiff neck is undressed and examined.
- Pain and stiffness may be the only symptoms of vertebral fracture or subluxation, which can occur without cord involvement – significant trauma merits A&E referral.
- Thunderclap headache preceding neck stiffness suggests subarachnoid haemorrhage: admit straight away.
- Consider serious bony pathology if pain and stiffness are relentless and wake the patient at night – especially if there are other worrying symptoms, or the patient has a past history of carcinoma.

NOTES:

STRIDOR IN CHILDREN

The GP overview

Acute stridor is a very frightening experience for both child and parents. The respiratory effort can lead to hyperventilation, making things worse. 'Difficult' or 'noisy' breathing in a child quite commonly leads to a request for an out-of-hours visit in winter. The usual cause is viral croup, producing mild, harmless stridor – but serious cases do occur. A calm exterior and a methodical approach are the keys to effective management.

Differential diagnosis

COMMON

- viral croup (laryngotracheobronchitis)
- acute epiglottitis
- acute laryngitis
- acute airways obstruction: foreign body (small toy, peanut)
- laryngeal paralysis (congenital: accounts for 25% of infants with stridor)

OCCASIONAL

- laryngomalacia
- laryngeal trauma
- bacterial tracheitis
- pseudomembranous croup (staphylococcal)
- upper airway burn

RARE

- laryngeal stenosis
- laryngeal tumours (papilloma, haemangioma) and mediastinal tumours
- laryngeal oedema (angioneurotic: oedema also present in other tissues)
- anomalous blood vessels, e.g. double aortic arch
- diphtheria
- retropharyngeal abscess

Ready reckoner

	Viral croup	Epiglottitis	Laryngitis	Obstruction	Laryngeal paralysis
Very sudden onset	No	Yes	No	Yes	No
Continuous stridor	Possible	Yes	No	Yes	Yes
Toxic and feverish	Possible	Yes	No	No	No
Drooling saliva	No	Yes	No	No	No
Very sore throat	No	Yes	No	Possible	No

Possible investigations

There are no investigations likely to be performed in primary care. The following might be performed in hospital: FBC (WCC raised in infection), lateral X-ray of pharynx (enlarged epiglottis in epiglottitis), CXR (may show foreign body, distal collapse or external compression of larynx or trachea) and laryngoscopy (for direct visualisation of the larynx).

TOP TIPS

- In practice, the first step is to exclude those conditions requiring immediate admission (epiglottitis or inhaled foreign body), leaving a probable diagnosis of viral croup. Management then depends on the child's general condition – in particular, the level of respiratory distress.
- Children with viral croup may have marked stridor and some recession when crying. It is reasonable to observe such children at home provided these signs disappear when the child is settled.
- When managing a child at home, make absolutely sure that the parents understand the signs of deterioration. If in doubt, arrange review.

- The toxic child with low-pitched stridor (often not marked), severe sore throat or difficulty in swallowing, and respiratory distress has epiglottitis until proved otherwise. Admit immediately and do not examine the throat (this can provoke respiratory obstruction).
- Restlessness, rising pulse and respiratory rate, increasing intercostal recession, fatigue and drowsiness are ominous signs: admit urgently regardless of precise diagnosis.
- Consider an inhaled foreign body if the onset is very sudden and there are no other symptoms or signs of respiratory infection.

NOSE

Blocked nose

Nosebleed

Runny/discharging nose

BLOCKED NOSE

The GP overview

This extremely common symptom is very familiar to all GPs. The most frequent cause, the common cold, is not included here, since nasal obstruction in itself is not usually the presenting symptom. The majority of causes of nasal obstruction are benign, but care should be taken to consider referral in those few cases that do not respond promptly to simple treatment.

Differential diagnosis

COMMON
- vasomotor rhinitis
- allergic rhinitis (seasonal and perennial)
- nasal polyps
- adenoidal hypertrophy (in children)
- nasal septal deviation (may affect 20% of adults)

OCCASIONAL
- overuse of over-the-counter nasal decongestants (rhinitis medicamentosa)
- chronic sinusitis
- papilloma
- trauma (including septal haematoma)
- foreign body (especially toddlers)

RARE
- iatrogenic, e.g. doxazosin
- carcinoma of nose and sinuses: squamous cell, adenocarcinoma
- other rare nasal tumours, e.g. melanoma, teratoma
- unilateral choanal atresia
- fibroangioma of puberty

Ready reckoner

	Vasomotor rhinitis	Allergic rhinitis	Adenoids	Polyps	Septal deviation
Sudden onset	Yes	Yes	No	No	No
Discharge	Yes	Yes	Possible	Possible	No
Sneezing	Possible	Yes	No	No	No
Unilateral	No	No	Possible	Possible	Yes
Previous trauma	No	No	No	No	Yes

Possible investigations

LIKELY: none.

POSSIBLE: sinus X-rays, allergy tests.

SMALL PRINT: FBC, adenoid X-ray, CT scan.

- ☑ Sinus X-rays may be helpful in confirming chronic sinusitis.
- ☑ Allergy tests may identify sensitivities to particular allergens.
- ☑ FBC: eosinophilia in allergic rhinitis (though rarely required for diagnosis).
- ☑ Adenoid X-ray: will confirm adenoidal hypertrophy.
- ☑ CT scan defines size and extent of nasopharyngeal carcinoma and sinus pathology.

TOP TIPS

- ☑ Nasal obstruction is usually the cause rather than the result of recurrent sinusitis. Dealing with the underlying problem may well relieve the sinusitis.
- ☑ Nasal allergy and polyps often coexist. It is worth trying medical treatment to relieve the symptoms before referring for polypectomy.
- ☑ Very sudden nasal blockage with profuse watery rhinorrhoea is likely to be caused by vasomotor rhinitis.
- ☑ If adenoidal nasal obstruction is present with possible hearing or speech difficulties, or possible sleep apnoea, refer with a view to adenoidectomy.

☑ Unilateral bloodstained discharge in an older patient with nasal blockage is sinister and suggests malignancy.

☑ Soft swelling either side of the septum following trauma suggests septal haematoma. This should be evacuated to reduce the risk of cartilage necrosis and infection.

☑ Check what over-the-counter nasal sprays the patient has been using, remembering the possibility of rhinitis medicamentosa.

☑ A toddler with a unilateral nasal blockage and foul-smelling discharge is likely to have a nasal foreign body.

NOTES:

NOSEBLEED

The GP overview

This is commonest in the very young and the very old. It may present routinely as a recurrent problem, or in the acute situation when the patient cannot control the bleeding. The latter cases usually result in trivial haemorrhage by clinical standards, but may create a disproportionate amount of alarm. Occasionally, a prolonged nosebleed can cause significant hypovolaemia, especially in the elderly.

Differential diagnosis

COMMON
- spontaneous (from Little's area; may be aggravated by nose-picking and sneezing)
- nasal infection and ulceration
- drugs, e.g. anticoagulants
- allergic rhinitis (and atrophic rhinitis)
- hypertension (often with atherosclerosis)

OCCASIONAL
- nasal sprays, e.g. corticosteroids
- septal granulomas and perforations
- severe liver disease
- tumours of nose and/or sinuses
- abnormal anatomy: septal deviation
- trauma: nasal fracture

RARE
- leukaemia
- thrombocytopenia
- coagulopathy: haemophilia, Christmas and von Willebrand's diseases
- vitamin deficiencies: C and K
- hereditary haemorrhagic telangiectasia

Ready reckoner

	Spontaneous	Hypertension	Infection	Drugs	Rhinitis
Recurrent	Possible	Yes	No	Yes	Yes
Generalised bruising	No	No	No	Yes	No
Discharge or crusting	No	No	Yes	No	No
Nasal congestion	No	No	Possible	No	Yes
Soreness/pain in nose	Possible	No	Yes	No	No

Possible investigations

LIKELY: none (INR if on warfarin).

POSSIBLE: FBC, clotting studies.

SMALL PRINT: LFT, sinus X-ray, CT scan.

- FBC: to check for thrombocytopenia or other signs of blood dyscrasia.
- LFT: severe (e.g. alcoholic) liver disease causes clotting problems.
- Raised INR may reflect severe liver disease or warfarin overdose.
- Further clotting studies: if disorders such as haemophilia or von Willebrand's disease are suspected.
- Sinus X-ray/CT scanning (usually secondary care): if tumour a possibility.

TOP TIPS

- Emergency calls for children with acute epistaxis can usually be dealt with by clear, calm and authoritative advice on the telephone. First-aid measures should also be advised in the elderly, but hospital referral may prove necessary, as the bleeding can be considerable and more difficult to stop.
- When children are presented in the surgery, establish any parental concerns. The main problem is often a fear of a blood disorder such as leukaemia rather than the inconvenience of the symptom itself.
- In young or middle-aged adults with recurrent bleeding and ulceration, consider cocaine abuse.
- Adults with recurrent epistaxis may well expect their blood pressure to be taken; either go ahead and take it, or, if the cause is obviously not hypertension, explain why there is no need.

☑ Severe nosebleed unresponsive to standard first-aid measures is best dealt with in hospital – especially in the elderly. Refer urgently to ENT or A&E.

☑ If recurrent nosebleeds with purpuric bruising, check FBC and coagulation screen urgently.

☑ Beware of recent onset of persistent unilateral bloodstained discharge and obstruction in the middle-aged and elderly. Carcinoma of the nose, nasopharynx or sinus is possible.

☑ Patients on warfarin should have an urgent INR and review of their dosage requirements.

NOTES:

RUNNY/DISCHARGING NOSE

The GP overview

Though not usually viewed as a significant symptom, this is very bothersome to those that suffer it. Many of the pathologies overlap with the causes of the 'Blocked nose' – please refer to this chapter too, as appropriate. The cause is rarely sinister, but referral for further assessment may be necessary if it persists in spite of treatment.

Differential diagnosis

COMMON
- URTI including common cold
- allergic rhinitis (seasonal or perennial)
- vasomotor rhinitis
- sinusitis
- infected nasal mucosal lesion (herpes simplex, impetigo)

OCCASIONAL
- polyps
- rhinitis medicamentosa
- cocaine abuse
- cluster headaches (though these will usually present with the pain)
- chemical irritation (smoke, fumes)
- nasal foreign body (usually seen in toddlers or children)
- drug side effects, e.g. α-blockers, calcium channel blockers

RARE
- malignancy
- CSF rhinorrhoea following head injury
- barotrauma ('sinus squeeze')
- *Corynebacterium diphtheriae* infection

Ready reckoner

	URTI	Allergic rhinitis	Vasomotor rhinitis	Acute sinusitis	Mucosal infection
Long history	No	Possible	Possible	No	No
Sneezing	Yes	Yes	Possible	Possible	Possible
Facial pain	Possible	No	No	Yes	No
Fever	Possible	No	No	Yes	No
Purulent discharge	Possible	No	No	Yes	Possible

Possible investigations

Usually none. Sinus X-rays, CT scan and allergy tests likely to be ordered by specialist after referral rather than in primary care.

TOP TIPS

- ☑ Use an auriscope with the largest available speculum to look into the nasal cavity – tell patients to hold their breath or the lens will steam up.
- ☑ Intermittently runny nose associated with a nasal obstruction that is dependent on position, e.g. disappears when lying down, suggests a single nasal polyp.
- ☑ Patients who describe their runny nose as 'just like turning on a tap' probably have vasomotor rhinitis.
- ☑ Remember to enquire about non-prescribed medication. Cocaine abuse, or the use of OTC sympathomimetic drops may be very relevant in making a diagnosis; and the response to any OTC treatments such as intranasal steroids might help guide diagnosis and further treatment.

- ☑ Intranasal foreign bodies are relatively common in toddlers – beware the unilateral foul-smelling nasal discharge in a child.
- ☑ A persistent bloodstained discharge requires investigation, especially if associated with unilateral nasal obstruction.
- ☑ Clear unilateral nasal discharge after direct trauma to the face may represent CSF leakage from an ethmoidal skull fracture. Occasionally this can present some time after the injury so beware the late presentation.

NOTES:

ORAL

Bad breath

Bleeding or painful gums

Mouth lumps and marks

Mouth ulcers

Painful tongue

BAD BREATH

The GP overview

This common symptom is usually caused by poor dental hygiene. As a presenting complaint it is seen far more often by dentists than GPs. It may be detected by a doctor examining a patient for an unrelated complaint, and rarely but significantly can herald serious pathology.

Differential diagnosis

COMMON
- ☑ poor dental hygiene
- ☑ heavy smoking
- ☑ gingivitis (including acute necrotising ulcerative gingivitis (ANUG), acute and chronic gingivitis)
- ☑ excess alcohol intake (acute and chronic)
- ☑ discharging dental abscess

OCCASIONAL
- ☑ ketohalitosis of starvation – especially in people using high-protein, high-fat, low-carbohydrate weight reduction diet regimens (and pre-operatively starved patients)
- ☑ drugs, e.g. disulfiram
- ☑ acute or chronic sinusitis
- ☑ subjectively perceived (non-existent) halitosis (sometimes a form of somatisation)
- ☑ GORD or acute gastroenteritis with reflux of gas

RARE
- ☑ bronchiectasis
- ☑ liver failure – hepatic foetor is said to smell like a freshly opened corpse; this is due to mercaptans in expired air
- ☑ true delusional subjective halitosis as part of psychiatric condition, e.g. severe depression with nihilism, psychotic illnesses
- ☑ rare oral or nasal conditions, e.g. pyogenic granuloma, discharging sinus from abscess

Ready reckoner

	Poor dental hygiene	Heavy smoking	Gingivitis	Excess alcohol	Dental abscess
Painful face/jaw	No	No	Possible	No	Yes
Bleeding gums	Possible	No	Yes	Possible	Possible
Facial swelling	No	No	No	No	Yes
Dental staining	Yes	Possible	Possible	No	Possible
Intoxication/stigmata of chronic alcohol abuse	No	No	No	Yes	No

Possible investigations

It is unlikely that the GP will initiate any investigations other than LFT if alcohol is a likely aetiology, or liver failure is suspected. CXR may be helpful if bronchiectasis is a possibility. Dentists may carry out the following investigations.

- Plaque and bleeding indexes – for oral hygiene.
- Basic periodontal examination – measurement of pocket depth between gums and teeth carried out with a specially marked probe.
- Oral pantomograph X-ray to investigate general state of teeth.

TOP TIPS

- If a dental cause is suspected, rather than telling the patient to make their own appointment with a dentist, give a short referral letter for them to hand over. This will ensure and record that you have carried out proper management and may speed things considerably for the patient.
- The vast majority of cases will involve oral hygiene. Be certain to exclude this, and other physical causes, before deciding that the halitosis is entirely subjective. As with other forms of somatisation, active management – with a psychiatric referral if necessary – is preferable to sending the patient away, only to return to make more appointments.
- If no obvious oral cause is found initially, extend the history and examination to include the respiratory and gastrointestinal systems.
- ANUG is a 'spot diagnosis' – the stench usually precedes the patient by some distance.

- ☑ In the absence of an obvious cause, do not neglect to examine the head and neck including the buccal cavity and nasal airway. Failure to do so could mean that a serious local cause is missed.
- ☑ Do not overlook alcohol abuse as a possible underlying cause.
- ☑ If the impact of the symptom seems out of all proportion to any objective sign of a problem, consider depression.

NOTES:

BLEEDING OR PAINFUL GUMS

The GP overview

The primary cause of this symptom is nearly always infection, usually because of poor dental hygiene: an endemic problem worldwide. Systemic problems may also cause gum pain or bleeding. While a dental referral is likely to be the end result, it is worth checking for general causes or easily remediable problems before directing the patient to the dentist.

Differential diagnosis

COMMON
- gingivitis/periodontal (gum) disease
- pregnancy gingivitis
- acute necrotising ulcerative gingivitis (ANUG): Vincent's stomatitis
- trauma: poorly fitting dentures
- drugs: warfarin overdosage, long-term phenytoin

OCCASIONAL
- aphthous ulceration
- acute herpetic gingivostomatitis (occasionally EBV)
- autoimmune disease: lichen planus, SLE and others
- oral neoplasia (commonest is SCC) (*Note:* may bleed but usually painless)
- blood dyscrasias (especially acute myeloid leukaemia)

RARE
- malabsorption (including scurvy)
- chemical poisoning: mercury, phosphorus, arsenic and lead
- hereditary haemorrhagic telangiectasia
- lymphangioma
- cavernous haemangioma

Ready reckoner

	Gingivitis	Pregnancy	ANUG	Trauma	Drugs
Swollen gums	Yes	Yes	Yes	Possible	Possible
Halitosis	Yes	No	Yes	No	No
Painful gums	Yes	No	Possible	Yes	No
Fever and malaise	No	No	Possible	No	No
Local lymphadenopathy	Possible	No	Yes	No	No

Possible investigations

LIKELY: none.

POSSIBLE: FBC.

SMALL PRINT: swab, INR, autoimmune screen, Paul–Bunnell test.

- ◪ FBC: to check for blood dyscrasias and malabsorption.
- ◪ Swab may help if obscure infective cause.
- ◪ Urgent INR if patient on warfarin.
- ◪ Paul–Bunnell test: EBV infection may cause gingivostomatitis.
- ◪ Autoimmune screen if autoimmune disease suspected.

TOP TIPS

- ◪ Patients with manifestly 'dental' problems may attend the GP because they view the doctor's service as cheaper or more accessible. Direct them firmly to the dentist to discourage inappropriate attendance in the future.
- ◪ Review the patient's medication – it is easy to overlook iatrogenic causes of gum soreness or bleeding.
- ◪ Patients with aphthous ulcers are likely to have read that their problem is associated with vitamin deficiencies or systemic illness. In primary care, it almost never is.
- ◪ Ulcerative gingivitis can often be diagnosed as soon as the patient walks into the consulting room, because of the characteristic odour.

- ◪ Children with primary attacks of herpetic gingivostomatitis can become quite ill and dehydrated. Consider early review or admission.
- ◪ Petechiae on the soft palate in conjunction with gingivostomatitis raise the possibility of EBV infection, acute leukaemia or scurvy.
- ◪ Enquire about skin problems elsewhere, or you may miss a significant diagnosis: SLE, pemphigus, pemphigoid, bullous erythema multiforme, epidermolysis bullosa and lichen planus can all affect the mouth.

MOUTH LUMPS AND MARKS

The GP overview

Mouth lumps and marks can be unfamiliar territory – partly because it is rarely an area of expertise for many GPs, and partly because many mouth problems are picked up by, or presented to, dentists in the first place. A proportion of patients will choose a GP as the first port of call, so a working knowledge of the area is useful.

Differential diagnosis

COMMON
- apical tooth abscess (gumboil)
- aphthous ulceration
- Fordyce spots (tiny white or yellow spots, on mucosa opposite molars and vermilion border of lips; they are sebaceous glands)
- oral candida infection
- mucocoele (solitary cystic nodule inside lip)

OCCASIONAL
- lichen planus
- trauma – bitten cheek
- ranula
- torus – benign maxillary or mandibular outgrowth of bone (very common but usually asymptomatic so not commonly seen)
- premalignant coloured areas: erythroplakia (red), leukoplakia (white), speckled leukoplakia (red and white), or verrucous leukoplakia
- geographical and hairy tongue
- tonsillar concretions
- other forms of oral ulceration (see Mouth ulcers, p. 356)

RARE
- malignancy – SCC or melanoma
- pachyderma oralis (from irritants)
- heavy metal poisoning (lead, bismuth, iron) – a dark line below the gingival margin
- cancrum oris

- sublingual dermoid cyst
- sublingual gland tumour
- pigmentation due to oral contraceptive pill – black or brown areas anywhere in the mouth
- Addison's disease – bluish hue opposite molars
- Peutz–Jeghers spots – brown spots on the lips
- telangiectasia – may be a sign of Osler–Weber–Rendu syndrome
- Stevens–Johnson syndrome

Ready reckoner

	Abscess	Ulcer	Fordyce spots	Candida	Mucocoele
Lesion tender	Yes	Yes	No	Possible	No
Flat lesion	No	Yes	No	Yes	No
Multiple lesions	No	Possible	Yes	Yes	No
White lesions	No	Yes	Possible	Yes	No
Lesion scrapes off	No	No	No	Yes	No

Possible investigations

LIKELY: none.

OCCASIONAL: FBC, ESR, CRP, ferritin, B_{12} and folate, fasting glucose or HbA1c, swab of lesion, HIV test.

SMALL PRINT: biopsy (performed at hospital).

- FBC, ESR, CRP and HIV are useful if immune deficiency (e.g. as a background to *Candida* infection) is suspected; FBC and ESR or CRP may be helpful in suspected malignancy too.
- Ferritin, B_{12} and folate deficiency is sometimes associated with oral aphthous ulceration – worth checking these in cases of recurrent or chronic ulceration (and see other possible investigations in Mouth ulcers, p. 356).
- Fasting glucose or HbA1c to investigate possible diabetes if candidal infection otherwise unexplained.
- Mouth swab to confirm candidal infection, though a diagnostic trial of treatment is often the practical first step.
- Biopsy: of suspicious lesions – this is inevitably performed in secondary care.

TOP TIPS

- Recurrent oral aphthous ulceration is a feature of a few systemic diseases (e.g. coeliac disease, Crohn's disease, Behçet's disease and AIDS) so be prepared to re-evaluate the history and widen the net of information gathering in repeat presentations.

- It is tempting to give antibiotics for a dental abscess, but the old surgical maxim 'if there's pus about, let it out' still holds true. Antibiotics may help reduce pain and surrounding infection but are only a temporary measure and may delay definitive treatment in those trying to avoid seeing a dentist, and increase the risk of complications. Encourage patients to see a dentist in the first place: offering a referral letter is helpful and may help to overcome any possible barrier to urgent access to a dentist at the dental reception desk.
- Always examine lumps by palpation from inside as well as outside the mouth. Wash latex gloves before the examination. Glove powder tastes foul!

Red flags

- Always refer the patient with permanent red or white buccal mucosal patches. Biopsy is indicated.
- If an ulcer fails to heal within a few weeks, especially if it is painless, refer for a specialist opinion as a suspected malignancy.
- Do not fail to examine regional lymph nodes. Enlarged nodes would be a significant finding, especially if they are non-tender and persistent.

NOTES:

MOUTH ULCERS

The GP overview

This symptom may often make a GP feel baffled – largely because it tends to be overlooked, or dealt with only briefly, during medical training. In fact common causes are simple to detect and treat, and it is clearly important to detect the occasional serious problem at an early stage. Examination could hardly be simpler, and a dentist may well have a clearer idea if referral is necessary in more obscure cases.

Differential diagnosis

COMMON
- trauma
- recurrent aphthous ulceration (RAU)
- acute necrotising ulcerative gingivitis (ANUG)
- thrush
- iron-deficiency anaemia (also vitamin B_{12} and folate deficiency)

OCCASIONAL
- Coxsackie virus: herpangina, hand, foot and mouth
- inflammatory bowel disease: ulcerative colitis and Crohn's disease
- coeliac disease
- herpes simplex and zoster
- glandular fever (EBV): infectious mononucleosis
- erosive lichen planus

RARE
- carcinoma: squamous cell, salivary gland
- autoimmune: Behçet's syndrome, pemphigoid, pemphigus, bullous erythema multiforme
- syphilitic chancre or gumma
- leukaemia, agranulocytosis (may be iatrogenic)
- tuberculosis
- HIV infection

Ready reckoner

	Trauma	RAU	ANUG	Thrush	Iron-deficiency anaemia
Usually in crops	No	Yes	Possible	Yes	Yes
White buccal plaques	No	No	No	Yes	No
Bleeding gums	No	No	Yes	No	No
Mucosal pallor	No	No	No	No	Yes
Recurrent	Yes	Yes	No	No	Possible

Possible investigations

LIKELY: FBC.

POSSIBLE: urinalysis, vitamin B_{12} and folate, coeliac screen.

SMALL PRINT: swab, autoantibody screen, syphilis and HIV serology, biopsy.

- FBC: essential basic investigation for anaemia and rarer blood dyscrasias.
- Urinalysis: check for glycosuria. Underlying diabetes may predispose to infective causes (especially *Candida*).
- Vitamin B_{12} and folate: to establish if underlying vitamin deficiency (especially if MCV raised).
- Coeliac screen: anti-endomysial and anti-gliadin antibodies suggest coeliac disease if positive.
- Swab: may help confirm doubtful diagnosis of ANUG – confirms presence of Vincent's organisms.
- Autoantibody screens and HLA tests may be useful if autoimmune causes are suspected.
- Syphilis or HIV serology: if syphilis or HIV are suspected.
- Biopsy: required in persistent ulcer of uncertain aetiology (secondary care investigation).

TOP TIPS

- Consider vitamin or iron deficiency, especially if the patient has glossitis and angular cheilitis as well as oral ulceration.
- The patient with sore, ulcerated gums and foul halitosis has ANUG; the smell is sometimes apparent as soon as the patient walks in.
- Patients with RAU often believe they are suffering from a vitamin deficiency; in fact, this is rarely the case, but be sure to broach this with them and consider a blood test as this may reinforce your reassurance.
- Enquire about skin problems elsewhere in an obscure case – this may give a clue to the precise diagnosis.
- Faucial ulceration and petechial haemorrhages of the soft palate and pharynx are likely to be caused by glandular fever.

☑ A solitary, persistent and often painless ulcer could be malignant – especially in smokers. Refer urgently to the oral surgeon for biopsy.

☑ Ask about bowel function: diarrhoea, abdominal pain and bloodstained stools with mucus suggest associated inflammatory bowel disease.

☑ Don't forget to enquire about medication: blood dyscrasias are a rare but significant side effect of some treatments (e.g. gold, carbimazole), and oral ulceration may be the first sign.

☑ Oral candidiasis is common in the debilitated and those with dentures, but much less so in the otherwise apparently fit. In the latter cases consider underlying problems such as immunosuppression or diabetes.

NOTES:

PAINFUL TONGUE

The GP overview

Pain in the tongue is usually caused by something immediately apparent on examination, but there are a few less obvious causes. This is something much more likely to be seen by a dentist, but is not strictly dental and therefore a working knowledge of the symptom is firmly within the GP remit.

Differential diagnosis

COMMON

- geographic tongue (benign migratory glossitis) – painful in some cases
- candidal infection (e.g. post-antibiotic, steroids and uncontrolled diabetes)
- trauma (bitten, burnt from hot food or drink)
- anaemia: iron, vitamins B_6 and B_{12}, and folate deficiency
- aphthous ulceration

OCCASIONAL

- viral infection, e.g. herpes simplex, hand, foot and mouth
- median rhomboid glossitis (superficial midline glossitis)
- burning mouth syndrome (also known as glossodynia)
- fissured tongue (doesn't commonly cause pain)
- glossopharyngeal neuralgia
- lichen planus

RARE

- carcinoma of the tongue
- Behçet's disease
- pemphigus vulgaris
- drugs, e.g. reserpine, mouthwashes, aspirin burns
- Moeller's glossitis

Ready reckoner

	Geographic	Candida	Trauma	Anaemia	Aphthous ulcer
Depapillation	Yes	Possible	No	Possible	No
White plaques	No	Possible	No	No	No
Localised pain	No	No	Yes	No	Yes
Pale mucosae	No	No	No	Yes	No
Recurrent	Yes	Possible	No	Possible	Yes

Possible investigations

LIKELY: FBC.

POSSIBLE: vitamin B_{12}, folate and ferritin assays, swab.

SMALL PRINT: biopsy.

- FBC initially to screen for anaemia.
- Vitamin B_{12}, folate and ferritin assays: if indicated by FBC.
- Swab of tongue may be helpful if appearance not obviously candidal.
- Biopsy of suspicious lesion to determine diagnosis (especially if possible carcinoma or pemphigus).

TOP TIPS

- Take note of self-medication. Aspirin sucked for toothache can cause a mucosal burn.
- A long history of soreness with spicy or bitter foods suggests geographic tongue or median rhomboid glossitis.
- A miserable, mildly febrile child with a painful tongue caused by numerous ulcers is likely to have a viral infection such as herpes simplex or hand, foot and mouth disease.
- Check the skin for other lesions in obscure cases – this may reveal the diagnosis (e.g. pemphigus, lichen planus).
- Patients with recurrent aphthous ulcers often erroneously believe they are deficient in vitamins – broach this concern with them.

Red flags

- If an ulcer in an adult fails to heal within a few weeks of presentation, refer urgently (though most oral neoplastic lesions are initially painless).
- The border of geographic tongue changes shape within weeks. This is not the case with more serious pathology.
- In candidal infections without an obvious cause, consider underlying diabetes or immunosuppression.
- Glossodynia characteristically produces burning pain on the tip of the tongue: a 'burner' is a dentist's heartsink and the symptom may signify underlying depression.

PELVIC

Acute pelvic pain

Chronic pelvic pain

Groin swellings

ACUTE PELVIC PAIN

The GP overview

This is nearly always seen in women rather than men. In its mildest form it is experienced universally at some time or other associated with periods, ovulation or sexual intercourse. In its severest form it is the commonest reason for urgent laparoscopic examination in the UK.

Differential diagnosis

COMMON
- acute pelvic inflammatory disease (PID)
- urinary tract infection (UTI)
- miscarriage
- ectopic pregnancy
- ovarian cysts: torsion, rupture

OCCASIONAL
- pelvic abscess (appendix, PID)
- endometriosis
- pelvic congestion (exacerbation of pelvic pain syndrome)
- prostatitis (men)
- functional (psychosexual origin)

RARE
- misplaced IUCD (perforated uterus)
- referred (e.g. spinal tumour, bowel spasm)
- proctitis
- invasive carcinoma of ovaries or cervix
- fibroid degeneration
- strangulated femoral or inguinal hernia

Ready reckoner

	PID	UTI	Miscarriage	Ectopic	Ovarian cyst
Abnormal vaginal bleeding	Possible	No	Yes	Possible	No
Purulent discharge PV	Yes	No	No	No	No
Fever	Yes	Yes	No	No	No
Palpable mass	No	No	Possible	No	Possible
Tender uterus PV	Yes	No	Possible	No	No

Possible investigations

LIKELY: HVS, cervical swab, urinalysis, MSU.

POSSIBLE: FBC, ESR/CRP, pregnancy test, ultrasound, laparoscopy (all usually arranged by hospital admitting team).

SMALL PRINT: none.

- ☑ Urinalysis: look for nitrites and pus cells to make diagnosis of UTI.
- ☑ MSU will confirm UTI and guide antibiotic treatment.
- ☑ HVS for bacteria including gonococcus and endocervical swab for *Chlamydia* if purulent discharge present.
- ☑ ESR/CRP: elevated in PID.
- ☑ Pregnancy test: positive in ectopic and miscarriage.
- ☑ FBC: raised WCC helps confirm PID and UTI if not being admitted. Also elevated in pelvic abscess.
- ☑ Urgent ultrasound helpful if miscarriage or ectopic pregnancy suspected.
- ☑ Cases referred to hospital are likely to undergo laparoscopy.

TOP TIPS

- ☑ In miscarriage, pain follows bleeding. In ectopic pregnancy, the sequence is usually reversed.
- ☑ Remember that there may be no bleeding with an ectopic pregnancy – or that the vaginal loss may be a light, blackish discharge.
- ☑ PV bleeding will cause haematuria on urinalysis. Only diagnose UTI if the symptoms are suggestive and urinalysis also shows nitrites and pus cells.

☑ Severe unilateral pain and tenderness PV around 6 weeks after last menstrual period (LMP) suggests ectopic pregnancy, even with no bleeding. Admit urgently.

☑ If PID does not settle within 48 hours of appropriate antibiotic treatment, consider abscess formation.

☑ Don't forget to check femoral and inguinal canals for a possible strangulated hernia.

NOTES:

CHRONIC PELVIC PAIN

The GP overview

Pelvic pain is defined as chronic if it has been present for three cycles or more. The difference between this and 'normal' period pain is one of intensity and duration. It is one of the commonest reasons for referral to a gynaecology clinic and for a woman to see her GP in the first place.

Differential diagnosis

COMMON
- endometriosis
- chronic pelvic inflammatory disease
- pelvic congestion
- irritable bowel syndrome
- physiological (mittelschmerz, primary dysmenorrhoea)

OCCASIONAL
- recurrent UTI
- musculoskeletal pain (back pain, pubic symphysis pain)
- uterovaginal prolapse
- benign tumours: ovarian cyst, fibroids
- chronic interstitial cystitis
- IUCD
- adhesions (from previous surgery)

RARE
- malignant tumours (ovary, cervix, bowel)
- diverticulitis
- lower colonic cancer
- inflammatory bowel disease
- subacute bowel obstruction

Ready reckoner

	Endometriosis	PID	Pelvic congestion	IBS	Physiological
Worse around period	Yes	Possible	Yes	Possible	Possible
Heavy periods	Yes	Yes	Yes	No	Possible
Altered bowel habit	No	No	No	Yes	No
Subfertility	Possible	Yes	No	No	No
Ovarian tenderness	Possible	Possible	Yes	No	No

Possible investigations

LIKELY: MSU, CA-125.

POSSIBLE: laparoscopy, ultrasound, HVS and cervical swab.

SMALL PRINT: FBC, ESR/CRP, bowel and back imaging.

- MSU detects UTI. Red cells alone may be present in interstitial cystitis.
- CA-125 – especially in women aged 50 or more to help rule out carcinoma of the ovary.
- FBC, ESR/CRP: WCC, ESR/CRP may be raised during exacerbation of chronic PID.
- HVS and cervical swab for *Chlamydia* may help in determining the infective agent in PID.
- Ultrasound is helpful if there is a palpable mass or if CA-125 is elevated.
- Laparoscopy is the investigation of choice for diagnosing PID, endometriosis and pelvic congestion.
- Further investigations, such as bowel and back imaging, might be undertaken by the specialist after referral.

TOP TIPS

- A 'forgotten' coil can cause cyclical pelvic pain.
- If the pain links with periods, establish whether it is primary or secondary dysmenorrhoea – the latter is far more likely to have a pathological cause.
- In some cases the diagnosis will remain obscure. Avoid colluding with obviously erroneous diagnoses and try to adopt a constructive approach without over-investigating the patient.
- Don't overlook non-gynaecological causes.
- Bloating is a very common gynaecological symptom, but is characteristic of IBS. A trial of antispasmodics may aid diagnosis.

- Women over 35 at first presentation and those with a mass should be referred for a gynaecological opinion.
- Misdiagnosis of PID without reliable evidence will delay the real diagnosis and lead to repeated courses of unnecessary antibiotics.
- Ovarian cancer nearly always presents late. Have a low threshold for investigation.
- Beware the diagnosis of endometriosis. Even if confirmed at laparoscopy, remember that many women with similar findings are asymptomatic. Discuss this openly with the patient – this will help prevent dysfunction if she does not improve with anti-endometriotic treatment.

NOTES:

GROIN SWELLINGS

The GP overview

Most causes of lumps in the groin are non-urgent. Many patients do not realise this, however – the development of a groin swelling often heralds an urgent appointment, either because the patient fears sinister pathology, or because the patient knows the diagnosis but erroneously perceives it as an emergency. GPs generally welcome the problem, as diagnosis and disposal are usually straightforward.

Differential diagnosis

COMMON
- sebaceous cyst
- palpable lymph nodes (LNs) – 'normal' or secondary to an infection
- inguinal hernia
- femoral hernia
- saphena varix

OCCASIONAL
- retractile testicle
- abscess (local)
- metastatic tumour (usually as skin-fixed lymphadenopathy)
- hydrocele of spermatic cord
- low appendix mass, pelvic/inguinal tumour
- lipoma

RARE
- abscess (psoas)
- lymphoma
- femoral artery aneurysm
- neurofibroma
- undescended or ectopic testis

Ready reckoner

	Sebaceous cyst	LNs	Inguinal hernia	Femoral hernia	Saphena varix
Reducible	No	No	Possible	Possible	Yes
Cough impulse	No	No	Yes	Possible	Yes
Palpable thrill on Valsalva manoeuvre	No	No	No	No	Yes
Fixed to skin	Yes	No	No	No	No
Originates above and medial to pubic tubercle	Possible	Possible	Yes	No	No

Possible investigations

LIKELY: none.

POSSIBLE: FBC, ESR/CRP, GUM screen.

SMALL PRINT: pelvic ultrasound.

- FBC and ESR/CRP useful if diffuse lymphadenopathy found, especially if no evidence of local cause or other significantly enlarged nodes found. Hb may be reduced and ESR/CRP elevated in malignancy; WCC and ESR/CRP elevated in abscess, infection and blood dyscrasias.
- Urethral, vaginal or endocervical swabs indicated if any associated discharge and/or suspicion of STD.
- Pelvic ultrasound useful if pelvic mass suspected.

TOP TIPS

- A large saphena varix can look very much like a small hernia. Try the Valsalva test (see Ready reckoner) and look for evidence of varicose veins.
- If the cause is local lymphadenopathy, look for local infective causes and don't forget to consider STDs.
- Don't be surprised to find no abnormality – normal groin nodes in a slim person, and a normally retractile testis can cause great anxiety in patients and parents.
- If the history suggests a hernia, but nothing is obvious on examination, get the patient to raise the intra-abdominal pressure with a vigorous cough or by raising the legs straight up while lying on the couch – and remember to examine the patient standing up, too.

Red flags

- ⌐ Femoral herniae (commoner in women) are at high risk of strangulation, so always refer.
- ⌐ Undescended testis in the adult carries a high risk of malignancy. If the testis is not descended by the age of 1 year, then operative intervention is indicated.
- ⌐ If lymphadenopathy is the cause, look elsewhere for abnormal lymph nodes and investigate or refer if any are found. Hard, skin-fixed nodes suggest metastatic malignancy – refer urgently.
- ⌐ An acutely painful and irreducible groin lump suggests a strangulated or incarcerated hernia. If in any doubt, refer for urgent surgical assessment.

NOTES:

PERIODS

Absent periods

Heavy periods

Irregular vaginal bleeding

Painful periods

ABSENT PERIODS

The GP overview

This symptom causes substantial anxiety in the sexually active woman: the first unexpectedly missed period suggests pregnancy; prolonged absence raises the concern that something is seriously amiss. In contrast, management is usually straightforward, and helped by acknowledging the anxiety.

Differential diagnosis

COMMON

- pregnancy
- physiological: rapid weight (10–15%) loss, and severe emotional stress
- menopause (including premature ovarian failure)
- polycystic ovary syndrome (PCOS)
- drugs: phenothiazines, metoclopramide, valproate, cytotoxics

OCCASIONAL

- hypo- and hyperthyroidism
- anorexia nervosa
- excessive exercise/training
- severe systemic illness of any kind
- contraception (progestogen-only pill, long-acting reversible contraception – common cause but rarely presented as a symptom)

RARE

- adrenal disorders: Addison's disease, Cushing's disease, congenital adrenal hyperplasia
- Sheehan's syndrome
- arrhenoblastoma, bilateral ovarian tumours
- prolactinoma, other pituitary tumours
- rare structural or chromosomal abnormalities (primary amenorrhoea)
- anterior pituitary failure (Simmonds's disease)

Ready reckoner

	Pregnancy	Weight loss	Menopause	Drugs	PCOS
Breast tenderness	Yes	No	No	No	No
Hot flushes	No	No	Yes	No	No
Obesity	No	No	No	No	Possible
Galactorrhoea	Yes	No	No	Possible	No
Depression	No	Possible	Possible	No	No

Possible investigations

LIKELY: pregnancy test.

POSSIBLE: FBC, U&E, TFT, FSH/LH, testosterone, prolactin, ultrasound.

SMALL PRINT: CT with or without other imaging.

- Pregnancy test whatever contraception is used: urinary HCG. Remember small false negative rate.
- FBC, U&E, TFT: to assess for general severe systemic illness, adrenal disorders and hypo- or hyperthyroidism.
- FSH, LH and testosterone: LH and testosterone high in PCOS, FSH very high in menopause.
- Prolactin levels high in prolactinoma and with some drugs (e.g. phenothiazines).
- Ultrasound useful to show multiple ovarian cyst formation and is a reliable check of pregnancy.
- Specialist will arrange CT or similar imaging if prolactinoma suspected.

TOP TIPS

- Amenorrhoea is common in young women, especially at times of stress; once pregnancy has been excluded and in the absence of any worrying symptoms or signs, only investigate if the problem persists beyond 6 months.
- It is important to confirm a possible diagnosis of premature menopause, as the patient will require hormone-replacement therapy (HRT).
- The same pathologies can cause both amenorrhoea and oligomenorrhoea, therefore take the same clinical approach to both.

☑ Do not accept too readily the claim that there is 'no chance of pregnancy'; if in any doubt, arrange a pregnancy test.

☑ Consider anorexia – an emaciated body may be well hidden under baggy clothing, and the disease often presents with the absence of periods.

☑ Early morning headache and visual disturbance associated with amenorrhoea suggest possible intracranial pathology – refer urgently.

☑ Before attributing amenorrhoea to weight loss, make sure that the weight loss itself hasn't been caused by thyrotoxicosis.

NOTES:

HEAVY PERIODS

The GP overview

This is a common presenting complaint. The average GP can expect about 100 women to consult each year for menstrual problems (female GPs rather more) and many of these will be for menorrhagia. Normal menstrual blood loss is 20–80 mL. In practice, measurement is not feasible, so the definition rests on what the woman reports, although some efforts can be made to establish whether or not the bleeding is 'excessive'.

Differential diagnosis

COMMON
- dysfunctional uterine bleeding (DUB)
- cervical or endometrial polyps
- endometriosis
- fibroids
- puberty and perimenopause

OCCASIONAL
- hypothyroidism (and hyperthryoidism)
- IUCD
- iatrogenic (contraceptive pill, HRT)
- cystic glandular hyperplasia (metropathia haemorrhagica)
- chronic PID

RARE
- adrenal disorders and hyperprolactinaemia
- liver disease, especially alcoholic
- clotting disorder
- endometrial carcinoma
- tuberculous endometritis

Ready reckoner

	DUB	Polyps	Endometriosis	Fibroids	Puberty/perimenopause
Long history	Possible	Possible	Possible	Possible	No
Long cycle	Possible	No	No	No	Possible
PVE: tender	No	No	Yes	No	No
Very painful periods	No	Possible	Yes	No	Possible
PVE: enlarged uterus	No	No	Possible	Yes	No

Possible investigations

LIKELY: FBC.

POSSIBLE: TFT, ESR/CRP, transvaginal ultrasound and, after referral, endometrial sampling and hysteroscopy.

SMALL PRINT: LFT, HVS, clotting studies, endocrine assays.

◪ FBC to check for anaemia and thrombocytopenia.
◪ Check possible thyroid dysfunction with TFT.
◪ ESR/CRP: elevated in PID.
◪ LFT: if clinical suspicion of liver disease.
◪ Clotting studies: if other history of abnormal bleeding or bruising.
◪ Transvaginal ultrasound useful for confirming fibroids and suggesting endometrial pathology.
◪ HVS very occasionally useful in chronic PID with discharge.
◪ Endocrine assays: for hyperprolactinaemia or adrenal disorders.
◪ Investigation after referral is likely to include endometrial sampling and/or hysteroscopy.

TOP TIPS

◪ Self-reporting of the heaviness of the menstrual flow is notoriously unreliable. Attempt an objective assessment by enquiring about the number of pads or tampons used, flooding, the presence of clots, and by checking an FBC for iron-deficiency anaemia.
◪ Establish the woman's agenda. This presentation may be the passport to a prescription (e.g. the contraceptive pill in a young woman) or to discussion of a specific anxiety (e.g. fears about possible cancer or a need for hysterectomy).
◪ Don't forget to enquire about a 'long-forgotten' coil.
◪ In a young woman who has painless heavy periods, is otherwise well and has a normal vaginal examination, it is reasonable to make a presumptive diagnosis of DUB and treat empirically.

- Establish whether the problem really is simply 'heavy periods'; if the bleeding is chaotic, or there is also intermenstrual or post-coital bleeding, the chances of a structural lesion are much higher – ensure the patient is appropriately investigated.
- Blood clots suggest significant bleeding; do not forget to arrange an FBC.
- Menorrhagia with secondary dysmenorrhoea, dyspareunia and pelvic tenderness on examination suggest endometriosis or chronic PID.

NOTES:

IRREGULAR VAGINAL BLEEDING

The GP overview

Irregular vaginal bleeding presents commonly in primary care – particularly to female GPs, as the patient will often anticipate a pelvic examination. This chapter covers all causes of this symptom throughout life including prepubertal, causes in early pregnancy and postmenopausal (causes in late pregnancy are not covered as they constitute a quite different clinical scenario). The key to appropriate management usually lies in a careful history.

Differential diagnosis

COMMON

- dysfunctional uterine bleeding (DUB)
- breakthrough bleeding (BTB) on contraceptive pills and long acting reversible contraception; also HRT
- cervical polyp or erosion
- cervicitis and PID
- post-menopausal atrophic vaginitis

OCCASIONAL

- endometrial polyps
- ovulatory bleeding (associated with mittelschmerz)
- hypothyroidism (and less commonly hyperthyroidism)
- perimenopause
- bleeding during early pregnancy (20% of all pregnancies in first trimester); also miscarriage, ectopic pregnancy

RARE

- uterine bleeding in the newborn
- carcinoma (ovary, fallopian tube, uterus, cervix and vagina)
- cystic glandular hyperplasia (metropathia haemorrhagica)
- pyometra
- hydatidiform mole (5% go on to chorionic carcinoma)

Ready reckoner

	DUB	BTB	Polyp/erosion	Cervicitis/PID	Atrophic vaginitis
Profuse bleeding	Possible	No	No	Possible	No
Painful periods	Possible	No	No	Yes	No
Discharge	No	No	Possible	Yes	Possible
Discomfort PV	No	No	No	Possible	Yes
Post-coital bleeding	No	No	Yes	Possible	Possible

Possible investigations

LIKELY: FBC, specialised gynaecological investigation (see below) for post-menopausal or intermenstrual bleeding.

POSSIBLE: HVS and endocervical swab, colposcopy, transvaginal ultrasound.

SMALL PRINT: TFT.

- FBC to check for anaemia in heavy bleeding. Raised WCC in PID.
- TFT: to check for possible thyroid dysfunction.
- HVS and endocervical swab: to attempt to establish pathogen in cervicitis and PID.
- Transvaginal ultrasound: to detect uterine and ovarian pathology, hydatidiform mole and to establish nature of problem in early pregnancy.
- Colposcopy: if significant cervical pathology suspected.
- Specialised gynaecological investigation (e.g. hysteroscopy and endometrial sampling): performed in secondary care, particularly for intermenstrual and postmenopausal bleeding.

TOP TIPS

- Try to distinguish between intermenstrual bleeding and irregular periods, as the likely causes are different (the former suggests a structural lesion, the latter is likely to be DUB). Simply asking the patient if the bleed feels like a period, with associated period-type symptoms, may help.
- Consider asking the patient to keep a menstrual diary. Very slight bleeding occurring consistently in mid-cycle with a slight pain and with no other worrying features suggests an ovulatory bleed.
- Remember that missed doses, diarrhoea and vomiting, and the first few months of treatment can cause breakthrough bleeding when using oral hormonal preparations. It is worth waiting a few more cycles before changing treatment.

Red flags

☑ Post-menopausal bleeding is always abnormal. Even if atrophic vaginitis is present, do not assume this is the cause: this symptom requires a full assessment.

☑ A very inflamed-looking cervix with a purulent discharge is likely to be caused by *Chlamydia* infection: consider referral to the local GUM clinic for further investigation and contact tracing.

☑ A 'recent' normal cervical smear can provide false reassurance; if the cervix looks suspicious, do not take another smear – remember, this is a screening, rather than diagnostic, test. Instead, refer urgently for colposcopy.

☑ Beware of 'breakthrough bleeding' in patients on hormonal contraception or HRT. If it persists, consider other causes and investigate or refer.

☑ Unilateral pelvic pain with vaginal bleeding within a fortnight of a missed period suggests an ectopic pregnancy. Admit urgently.

NOTES:

PAINFUL PERIODS

The GP overview

Painful periods are extremely common: 50% of women in the UK complain of moderate pain, and 12% suffer severe, disabling pain. Primary dysmenorrhoea is pain with no organic pathology, usually starting when ovulatory cycles begin. Secondary dysmenorrhoea is associated with pelvic pathology, and appears later in life.

Differential diagnosis

COMMON

- primary dysmenorrhoea
- endometriosis
- chronic PID
- IUCD
- pelvic pain syndrome ('venous congestion')

OCCASIONAL

- retroverted uterus
- cervicitis
- chocolate cyst of ovary
- endometrial polyp

RARE

- uterine malformation
- imperforate hymen
- uterine hypoplasia
- cervical stenosis
- psychogenic

Ready reckoner

	Primary	Endometriosis	PID	Pelvic congestion	IUCD
During first few days of period only	Yes	No	No	No	No
Deep dyspareunia	No	Yes	Yes	Yes	No
Colicky pain	Yes	No	No	No	Yes
Begins in adulthood	No	Yes	Yes	Yes	Yes
Enlarged uterus O/E	No	Possible	No	Possible	No

Possible investigations

LIKELY: none.

POSSIBLE: FBC, ESR/CRP, HVS and endocervical swab, ultrasound, laparoscopy.

SMALL PRINT: none.

- FBC for anaemia if periods also heavy. WCC and ESR/CRP raised in PID.
- HVS and endocervical swab for *Chlamydia* if vaginal discharge present – may help establish pathogen in chronic PID.
- Ultrasound helpful to define uterine enlargement or other abnormalities and to detect ovarian cysts.
- Laparoscopy is the usual investigation after referral to secondary care: will make diagnosis of PID and endometriosis.

TOP TIPS

- Explore the patient's agenda: young adolescents may use the symptom of painful periods as a passport symptom to obtain a prescription for the contraceptive pill.
- Beware of the diagnosis of endometriosis. Even if detected laparoscopically, this may not be the actual cause of the patient's pain (endometriosis is often asymptomatic). Unless it is explained that the treatment offered is not necessarily a panacea, the patient is likely to get frustrated at the apparent lack of progress.
- A long-forgotten IUCD can be a cause of dysmenorrhoea. Enquire specifically about this possibility – and check the notes too.
- Explain to patients early on in your management that a precise organic diagnosis isn't always possible; this will help maintain a good doctor–patient relationship, which will facilitate the subsequent unravelling of any significant underlying psychological problems.

- The chances of organic pathology are greater if the patient has secondary dysmenorrhoea which is severe enough to disturb sleep.
- Half of women who undergo laparoscopy for secondary dysmenorrhoea have no obvious organic pathology. Consider psychological problems and avoid over-investigating and over-referring – a number of these women end up having surgery (e.g. TAH) but even then continue to have pain.
- Consider other pathologies if the patient presents acutely with a self-diagnosis of 'severe period pain': non-gynaecological causes of pelvic pain such as appendicitis, renal colic or UTI may occur at the expected time of the period.
- While painful periods are depressing, true clinical depression may lower the pain threshold of an otherwise normal woman and should not be missed.

NOTES:

SKIN

Blisters (vesicles and bullae)

Erythema

Macules

Nodules

Papules

Purpura and petechiae

Pustules

Scales and plaques

BLISTERS (VESICLES AND BULLAE)

The GP overview

Blisters are skin swellings containing free fluid. Up to 5 mm they are called vesicles, larger than 5 mm they are called bullae. The fluid can be lymph, serum, extracellular fluid or blood. Some conditions cause both kinds of blister, but others mainly one or other type. Pustules are dealt with elsewhere (see p. 403).

Differential diagnosis

COMMON
- trauma: skin friction, burns (thermal and chemical), insect bites
- herpes simplex
- herpes zoster
- childhood viruses: hand, foot and mouth disease, chickenpox
- eczema (pompholyx and other acute eczemas)

OCCASIONAL
- pemphigus and pemphigoid
- dermatitis herpetiformis
- secondary to leg oedema (various causes)
- bullous impetigo
- drug reactions, e.g. ACE inhibitors, penicillamine, barbiturates
- erythema multiforme

RARE
- pemphigoid (herpes) gestationis
- porphyria
- toxic epidermal necrolysis (Lyell's syndrome)
- epidermolysis bullosa
- allergic vasculitis

Ready reckoner

	Trauma	Herpes simplex	Herpes zoster	Childhood viruses	Eczema
Vesicles	No	Yes	Yes	Yes	Possible
Bullae	Yes	Possible	Possible	No	Possible
Recurrent	No	Yes	No	No	Yes
Unilateral	Possible	Possible	Yes	No	Possible
Painful	Yes	Yes	Yes	No	Possible

Possible investigations

There are unlikely to be any investigations that will prove useful in primary care. Usually, the problem is either self-limiting or the cause obvious; in obscure cases, referral may result in skin biopsy to establish the diagnosis. Patch testing may also be useful to identify possible allergens in contact dermatitis, especially if occupational.

TOP TIPS

- Herpes zoster involving the ophthalmic division of the trigeminal nerve will affect the eye in about 50% of cases. The likelihood is increased if there are blisters on the side of the nose. Ensure that the patient knows to seek help urgently if the eye becomes red or painful, or there is blurring of vision.
- In uncomplicated herpes zoster, explain the natural history of the condition to the patient, resolving any worries (old wives' tales abound) and warning about the possibility of post-herpetic neuralgia.
- Follow up unexplained rashes. The bullae of pemphigoid, for example, may be preceded by itching, erythema and urticaria by several weeks.

Red flags

- Herpes simplex and varicella zoster infections can become severe and disseminated in the immunosuppressed: admit. Similarly, herpes simplex can result in a serious reaction (Kaposi's varicelliform eruption) in patients with atopic eczema.
- Pregnant women with chickenpox are at significant risk of severe varicella pneumonia; there are also risks to the foetus. Follow the detailed guidance in the 'Green Book' (*Immunisation against Infectious Disease*, Her Majesty's Stationery Office) when dealing with pregnant women who have been in contact with chickenpox.
- Toxic epidermal necrolysis (scalded skin syndrome) can develop rapidly in infants and children, causing serious illness. Admit urgently if you suspect this diagnosis.
- Pemphigus is a serious condition affecting a younger age group (usually middle-aged) than pemphigoid. Inpatient care is usually required.

ERYTHEMA

The GP overview

Erythema is a reddening of the skin due to persistent dilation of superficial blood vessels, and can be local or generalised. It is distinguished from flushing (see p. 197) by its permanence: flushing is transient.

Differential diagnosis

COMMON

- cellulitis
- gout
- burns: thermal, chemical, sunburn
- toxic erythema: drugs (e.g. antibiotics, NSAIDs), bacteria (e.g. scarlet fever), viruses (e.g. measles, slapped cheek syndrome)
- rosacea

OCCASIONAL

- palmar erythema, e.g. pregnancy, liver disease, thyrotoxicosis
- phototoxic reaction to drugs, e.g. phenothiazines, tetracyclines, diuretics
- 'deck-chair legs' (prolonged immobility)
- erythema multiforme (various causes)
- systemic lupus erythematosus (erythematous, photosensitive butterfly rash)
- erythema ab igne (reticulate pattern)

RARE

- fixed drug eruption
- livedo reticularis: connective tissue disease
- seroconversion rash of HIV
- erythema nodosum: sarcoidosis, streptococci, tuberculosis, drugs
- erythema induratum (Bazin's disease: tuberculosis)
- erythema chronicum migrans: Lyme disease

Ready reckoner

	Cellulitis	Gout	Burns	Toxic erythema	Rosacea
Fever	Yes	Possible	No	Possible	No
Pustules	No	No	No	No	Yes
Periarticular	Possible	Yes	Possible	Possible	No
Blisters	Possible	No	Possible	Possible	No
Widespread	No	No	Possible	Yes	No

Possible investigations

LIKELY: uric acid (if possible gout).

POSSIBLE: FBC, ESR/CRP, LFT, TFT.

SMALL PRINT: autoimmune studies, serology, CXR, ASO titre.

- FBC/ESR/CRP: WCC and ESR/CRP raised in significant infection; Hb may be reduced (normochromic normocytic) in connective tissue disorder.
- Autoimmune studies: if connective tissue disorder a possibility.
- Serology: may help if suspect infective cause for erythema multiforme; also useful in assessing immune status in a pregnant woman exposed to slapped cheek syndrome, and in diagnosis of HIV infection and Lyme disease.
- Uric acid: to confirm clinical suspicion of gout (when attack has subsided) especially if considering allopurinol.
- LFT, TFT: if palmar erythema present in non-pregnant patient – to detect alcohol excess or hyperthyroidism.
- Other investigations for erythema nodosum: if a non-drug cause is possible, investigations likely to include CXR (for TB, sarcoidosis) and ASO titre (for streptococcal infection).

TOP TIPS

- Toxic erythema caused by drugs tends to be itchy; if due to infection, it does not irritate but is accompanied by fever.
- Remember that there is often a delay before a drug causes toxic erythema – therefore, symptoms may only appear after a course of treatment (especially antibiotics) has been completed.
- 'Deck-chair legs' is erythema of the lower legs, sometimes with oedema and blistering, in the immobile. It tends to be mistakenly diagnosed as persistent or recurrent cellulitis.
- A violent local erythema, rapidly darkening and blistering and recurring at the same site, suggests a fixed drug eruption.

Red flags

- Erythema nodosum and multiforme may be caused by significant disease, including, very occasionally, malignancy. If the patient is generally unwell or has other significant symptoms, investigate urgently or refer.
- Take a travel history: Lyme disease is endemic in forested areas. If not diagnosed and treated early, it can have significant complications.
- Erythema multiforme with blistering and ulceration of the mucous membranes is Stevens–Johnson syndrome. Though rare, it is a very serious illness requiring urgent hospital treatment.
- Enquire about joint symptoms: many causes of erythema (e.g. erythema multiforme, butterfly rash, livedo reticularis) are linked to a connective tissue isorder.
- Remember to take a drug history, including over-the-counter medications. This may reveal the underlying cause in toxic erythema, erythema nodosum and multiforme, and phototoxicity.
- Remember that parvovirus can cause serious problems in pregnancy – check serology in women with suggestive symptoms, or exposure to a case.

NOTES:

MACULES

The GP overview

A macule is a flat, demarcated, abnormally coloured area of skin of any size. It may be red (e.g. drug eruption), dark red (e.g. purpura), brown (e.g. a flat mole) or white (e.g. pityriasis versi-color). Purpura is described elsewhere (see p. 400). There is some crossover between erythema (see p. 390) and red macules.

Differential diagnosis

COMMON
- drug reaction/allergy
- flat mole (junctional naevus)
- non-specific viral exanthem
- sun-induced freckles (including solar lentigines)
- chloasma

OCCASIONAL
- measles and rubella
- post-inflammatory hypo- or hyperpigmentation
- *café au lait* spot (creamy brown) and Mongolian spot (brown or slate-grey)
- Berloque dermatitis (brown: chemical photosensitisation, e.g. bergamot oil)
- depigmentation: vitiligo, pityriasis versicolor, pityriasis alba

RARE
- infections: macular syphilide, tuberculoid leprosy, typhoid (rose spots in 40%)
- Albright's syndrome
- neurofibromatosis (associated with more than six *café au lait* spots)
- pathological freckles: Hutchinson's freckle, Peutz–Jeghers syndrome
- naevus anaemicus (permanent vasoconstriction due to neurovascular abnormality)

Ready reckoner

	Drug reaction	Flat mole	Viral	Freckles	Chloasma
Itching and burning	Yes	No	No	No	No
Variable pigmentation	No	Yes	No	Possible	Possible
Red	Yes	No	Yes	No	No
<0.5 cm diameter	Possible	Possible	Possible	Yes	No
Symmetrical, muzzle area	No	No	No	No	Yes

Possible investigations

There are very few relevant investigations to consider and they would be required only exceptionally, as the diagnosis is usually clinical: skin scrapings for mycology or fluorescence under Wood's light may help in the diagnosis of pityriasis versicolor; acute and convalescent serum samples may confirm rubella; serology for syphilis may be appropriate with an unusual macular rash; and very occasionally, a skin biopsy may be required to clinch an obscure diagnosis.

TOP TIPS

- ▱ A drug eruption can take 2 weeks to appear from the time of the first dose – so don't be misled by the fact that a course of antibiotics may have been completed some days before the related drug rash develops.
- ▱ Pityriasis versicolor may be misdiagnosed as vitiligo. If in doubt, take scrapings for mycology or examine under Wood's light.
- ▱ Odd lines of hyperpigmentation on the sides of the neck are likely to be Berloque dermatitis – a photosensitive rash caused by oil of bergamot, present in perfumes.

- ▱ Hutchinson's freckle is a giant, variegated freckle, seen in elderly sun-exposed skin. There is a high risk of malignant change, so refer.
- ▱ Rubella is rare, but may become commoner as a result of media coverage of 'immunisation scares'. Establish whether or not a young woman presenting with a rubella-type rash is pregnant – if she is, confirm her rubella status.
- ▱ A child with very many freckles on and around the lips may have Peutz–Jeghers syndrome. This is associated with small bowel polyposis.
- ▱ Vitiligo tends to have a poor prognosis in Caucasians, especially if it is widespread and affecting lips and extremities.

NODULES

The GP overview

Skin nodules are larger than papules – more than 5 mm diameter. However, their depth is more significant clinically than their width. Some are free within the dermis; others are fixed to skin above or subcutaneous tissue below. The causes are various; the patient is usually concerned about the cosmetic appearance or malignant potential.

Differential diagnosis

COMMON
- sebaceous cyst
- lipoma
- basal cell carcinoma (BCC)
- warts
- xanthoma

OCCASIONAL
- dermatofibroma (histiocytoma)
- squamous cell carcinoma
- nodulocystic acne
- kerato-acanthoma
- gouty tophi
- chondrodermatitis nodularis chronica helicis
- rheumatoid nodules and Heberden's nodes
- pyogenic granuloma

RARE
- malignant melanoma (becoming more common in the UK)
- vasculitic: erythema nodosum, nodular vasculitis, polyarteritis nodosa
- atypical infections (e.g. leprosy, treponema, lupus vulgaris, fish tank and swimming pool granuloma, actinomycosis)
- lymphoma and metastatic secondary carcinoma
- sarcoidosis
- pretibial myxoedema

Ready reckoner

	Xanthoma	Sebaceous cyst	BCC	Wart	Lipoma
Reddish-brown	Yes	No	Yes	No	No
Central punctum	No	Yes	No	No	No
Characteristic distribution	Yes	No	Yes	No	No
Normal skin surface	No	Yes	No	No	Yes
Multiple	Yes	No	Possible	Possible	Possible

Possible investigations

LIKELY: none (skin biopsy or cytology if doubt about the lesion or clinical diagnosis of possible carcinoma).

POSSIBLE: lipid profile, FBC, ESR/CRP, urate, rheumatoid factor, urinalysis.

SMALL PRINT: TFT, Kveim test, further investigations guided by clinical picture (see below).

- Excision biopsy is the definitive investigation for achieving a diagnosis; cytology from skin scrapings can be used to diagnose BCC.
- Lipid profile: xanthomata require a full lipid profile to define the underlying hyperlipidaemia.
- Urinalysis: if suspect inflammatory or vasculitic skin lumps, as may reveal proteinuria if associated with systemic and renal disorders.
- FBC and ESR/CRP: ESR/CRP raised in inflammatory disorders and malignancy; may also reveal anaemia of chronic disease or malignancy (including lymphoma).
- Check urate if gouty tophi are clinically likely.
- Rheumatoid factor: nodules are usually associated with positive rheumatoid factor.
- TFT: to diagnose Graves's disease with pretibial myxoedema.
- Kveim test: may contribute to a diagnosis of sarcoidosis.
- Further investigations according to clinical picture: some lesions, such as erythema nodosum, may require further investigation to establish the underlying cause; histological confirmation of skin secondaries may similarly require further assessment, although the overall condition of the patient may mean this is a futile exercise.

TOP TIPS

- Look at the lesion under the magnifying glass – this may reveal suspicious signs such as ulceration or a rolled, pearly edge.
- In uncertain cases which do not require urgent attention, record your findings carefully (including precise dimensions) and review in a month or two.
- Stoical patients may underestimate the significance of a suspicious lesion, particularly if you discover it during a routine examination – if you are referring them for biopsy, impress upon them the need to attend their appointment.

▨ Establish the patient's concern, which will usually centre on worries about cosmetic appearance or cancer. This will result in a more functional consultation and a more satisfied patient.

▨ Night sweats and itching with skin nodules raises the suspicion of lymphoma. Examine lymph nodes, liver and spleen carefully.

▨ The elderly patient complaining of a lesion in a sun-exposed area which 'just won't heal' may well have a squamous or basal cell carcinoma.

▨ The appearance of a nodule in a mole is highly significant and requires referral.

▨ A patient with nodulocystic acne requires referral to a dermatologist for possible treatment with 13-*cis*-retinoic acid.

▨ The unwell middle-aged or elderly patient who develops bizarre and widespread skin nodules over a period of a few weeks probably has an underlying carcinoma.

NOTES:

PAPULES

The GP overview

Papules are solid, circumscribed skin elevations up to 5 mm in diameter. If they are larger, they are called nodules – these are dealt with elsewhere (see p. 395). (Clearly, many nodules start life as a papule; to avoid confusion, if they are generally 'nodular' by the time they present to the GP, then they are dealt with in that section, and not repeated here.) They are usually round but the shape, and the colour, may vary. They may be transitional lesions, e.g. becoming vesicular, or about to ulcerate.

NOTE: there are more causes of papules than can be listed here. This is a sensible selection.

Differential diagnosis

COMMON
- acne
- scabies
- viral wart and molluscum contagiosum
- Campbell de Morgan spot
- skin tag

OCCASIONAL
- viral illness
- milia
- insect bites
- early seborrhoeic wart
- xanthomata
- guttate psoriasis
- pityriasis lichenoides chronica, lichen planus
- prickly heat
- keratosis pilaris

RARE
- malignant melanoma, early basal cell carcinoma, Kaposi's sarcoma
- Darier's disease
- acanthosis nigricans
- pseudoxanthoma elasticum
- tuberous sclerosis

Ready reckoner

	Acne	Scabies	Viral wart	C. de M. spot	Skin tag
Itchy	No	Yes	No	No	No
Characteristic distribution	Yes	Yes	No	Yes	No
Red	Yes	Yes	No	Yes	No
Associated lesions	Yes	Yes	No	No	No
History of contact	No	Yes	Possible	No	No

Possible investigations

In practice, very few investigations are needed with this presentation: a lipid screen is required in the presence of xanthomata; genital warts require referral for screening for other STDs; thorough investigation may be needed in the very rare case where underlying malignancy is possible (e.g. acanthosis nigricans); and obscure rashes or solitary papules may occasionally require excision biopsy for a definitive diagnosis.

TOP TIPS

- ◪ Bear in mind that skin cancer is usually uppermost in the patient's mind, especially in subacute or chronic cases – so provide appropriate reassurance.
- ◪ In obscure solitary lesions, record clinical findings carefully and arrange to review in due course.
- ◪ Itchy, asymmetrical grouped papules are likely to be insect bites, although the patient may take some convincing!

- ◪ An enlarging dark blue or blue-black papule may be a malignant melanoma, blue naevus or Kaposi's sarcoma. Refer for urgent opinion.
- ◪ Brown, skin-coloured papules crowded around the nose of a child may be tuberous sclerosis. This can be associated with serious systemic pathology so refer for expert opinion.
- ◪ An intensely itchy papular rash which is worse at night and has no other obvious cause is likely to be scabies, even if scabetic burrows are not evident – treat on suspicion.

NOTES:

PURPURA AND PETECHIAE

The GP overview

Purpura are reddish-purple lesions which do not blanch with pressure. When less than 1 cm in diameter, they are called petechiae; if larger, they are known as ecchymoses. The problem often presents as 'bruising easily' – a common 'while I'm here' complaint in primary care. Most cases are normal, with causative minor trauma simply being forgotten or unnoticed.

Differential diagnosis

COMMON
- trauma
- senile purpura
- liver disease (especially alcoholic cirrhosis)
- increased intravascular pressure, e.g. coughing, vomiting, gravitational
- drugs, e.g. steroids, warfarin, aspirin

OCCASIONAL
- vasculitis, e.g. Henoch–Schönlein purpura, connective tissue disorders
- thrombocytopenia, e.g. idiopathic thrombocytopenia purpura (ITP), bone marrow damage (e.g. lymphoma, leukaemia, cytotoxics), aplastic anaemia
- renal failure
- infective endocarditis

RARE
- paraproteinaemias, e.g. cryoglobulinaemia
- inherited clotting disorders, e.g. haemophilia, Christmas disease, von Willebrand's disease
- infections, e.g. meningococcal septicaemia, Rocky Mountain spotted fever
- vitamin C and K deficiency
- disseminated intravascular coagulation (DIC)
- congenital vessel wall abnormalities, e.g. Ehlers–Danlos syndrome

Ready reckoner

	Trauma	Senile purpura	Liver disease	Increased IV pressure	Drugs
Tender bruising	Yes	No	No	No	No
Spontaneous	No	Possible	Yes	No	Yes
Widespread	No	Yes	Yes	No	Yes
Recurrent	No	Yes	Yes	No	Possible
Petechial	Possible	No	No	Yes	Possible

Possible investigations

LIKELY: FBC, ESR/CRP, INR (if on warfarin).

POSSIBLE: LFT, U&E, coagulation screen, plasma electrophoresis.

SMALL PRINT: autoimmune testing, further hospital investigations (see below).

- ◪ FBC, ESR/CRP: FBC may reveal thrombocytopenia or evidence of blood dyscrasia. ESR/CRP and WCC may be raised in blood dyscrasia, connective tissue disorder and infection.
- ◪ LFT, U&E: for underlying liver or renal disease.
- ◪ INR: if on warfarin.
- ◪ Autoimmune testing: if possible connective tissue disease causing vasculitis.
- ◪ Coagulation screen: to test haemostatic function, e.g. bleeding time, prothrombin time, activated partial thromboplastin time.
- ◪ Plasma electrophoresis: for hypergammaglobulinaemia, paraproteinaemia and cryoglobulinaemia.
- ◪ Further investigations (usually secondary care): to investigate underlying cause, e.g. skin biopsy to confirm vasculitis, bone marrow biopsy if possible marrow infiltrate.

TOP TIPS

- ◪ Multiple bruises of varying ages on the legs of young children who are otherwise well and have no other stigmata of clotting disorder or abuse are likely to be non-pathological.
- ◪ Senile purpura should be easy to diagnose from the history and examination. Reassurance, rather than investigation, is required.
- ◪ A few petechiae on or around the eyelids of a well child can be caused by vigorous coughing or vomiting. If the history is clear, explain the cause to the parents – but emphasise that the appearance of an identical rash elsewhere requires urgent attention.
- ◪ The distribution of purpura can give useful clues to the diagnosis. On the legs, platelet disorders, paraproteinaemias, Henoch–Schönlein purpura or meningococcal septicaemia are likely; lesions on the fingers and toes indicate vasculitis; and senile and steroid purpura tend to affect the back of the hands and arms.
- ◪ Purpura caused by vasculitis tend to be raised palpably above the skin.

□ Remember that the rash of meningococcal septicaemia can appear before a child is obviously systemically unwell. If there is any suspicion that this might be the diagnosis, give parenteral penicillin and admit immediately.

□ The absence of a family history does not exclude a significant inherited bleeding disorder: these disorders can arise spontaneously.

□ Take very seriously the pale patient with purpura: a bone marrow problem is likely. Arrange an urgent FBC or admit.

□ Always do a full surface examination of a child with bruising, not forgetting the anogenital area. Keep non-accidental injury in mind.

□ Never give an IM injection if a serious bleeding disorder is suspected.

NOTES:

PUSTULES

The GP overview

Pustules are raised lesions less than 0.5 cm in diameter containing a yellow fluid. They signify infection to most people, and will often present in an urgent appointment, as they are likely to have appeared suddenly. Patients will often expect antibiotic treatment. This will not always be necessary, so be prepared to offer a clear explanation and an appropriate alternative.

Differential diagnosis

COMMON
- impetigo
- other staphylococcal infections, e.g. early boils, folliculitis, sycosis barbae
- herpes simplex and zoster
- acne vulgaris
- rosacea

OCCASIONAL
- perioral dermatitis
- hidradenitis suppurativa (axillae and groins)
- candidiasis (satellite vesicopustules around moist eroded patch)
- pustular psoriasis (palmar and plantar commoner than generalised pustular psoriasis of von Zumbusch)

RARE
- dermatitis herpetiformis
- Behçet's syndrome
- viral: cowpox and orf (*Note:* chickenpox is vesicular, not pustular)
- hot tub folliculitis (superficial *Pseudomonas* infection)
- drug induced

Ready reckoner

	Impetigo	Other staphylococci	Herpes simplex or zoster	Acne vulgaris	Rosacea
Grouped or single	Possible	Possible	Yes	No	No
Staphylococcal	Yes	Yes	No	No	No
Recurrent	No	Possible	Possible	Yes	Yes
Affects eye	No	No	Possible	No	Possible
Tingling before lesion	No	No	Yes	No	No

Possible investigations

There are very few investigations likely to prove useful or necessary in primary care. The presence of widespread or recurrent candidal or staphylococcal lesions might necessitate a urinalysis or blood sugar to exclude diabetes; a swab of pus may help confirm a clinically suspected infective agent; and in very obscure cases, a skin biopsy might prove helpful.

TOP TIPS

- Take time to explain to the patient the nature of the problem in recurrent staphylococcal infections. Exclude diabetes, check carrier sites and reassure that the patient's 'hygiene' is not in question. A prolonged course of antibiotics may be helpful.
- Check self-treatment in rosacea and perioral dermatitis. Treatment with OTC topical steroids will exacerbate the problem. Warn the patient that the condition may worsen before it improves on withdrawal of this inappropriate treatment.
- Papules and pustules around the mouth and eyes, often with a halo of pallor around the lip margin, are caused by perioral dermatitis. Treat with antibiotics, not topical steroids.

- Widespread, severe and recurrent staphylococcal lesions suggest diabetes or possible immunosuppression.
- Localised pustular psoriasis can be very resistant to standard treatments, so have a low threshold for referral. The very rare generalised form can make the patient dangerously ill: admit urgently.
- Remember that herpes simplex or zoster infections in the immunocompromised can become disseminated and severe.
- Ocular problems in rosacea can be complicated and troublesome: refer to an ophthalmologist.

SCALES AND PLAQUES

The GP overview

Skin scales represent an abnormally fast piling up of keratinised epithelium. Scales and plaques are common at all ages and have a variety of causes. The presentation will centre on cosmetic appearance, itching, fears about serious disease or a combination of these.

Differential diagnosis

COMMON

- psoriasis
- eczema (in all its various forms)
- fungal infections (e.g. scalp, body, feet)
- seborrhoeic dermatitis
- seborrhoeic keratosis

OCCASIONAL

- lichen simplex
- lichen planus (usually scaly only on legs)
- solar keratosis
- pityriasis versicolor and rosea
- juvenile plantar dermatosis
- guttate psoriasis (scaly papules)

RARE

- malignancy: Bowen's disease and mycosis fungoides (cutaneous T-cell lymphoma)
- drug induced (e.g. β-blockers and carbamazepine)
- ichthyosis (various forms)
- keratoderma blenorrhagica (part of Reiter's syndrome)
- pityriasis lichenoides chronica
- secondary syphilis

Ready reckoner

	Psoriasis	Eczema	Fungal	Seborrhoeic dermatitis	Seborrhoeic keratosis
Plaque	Yes	Possible	No	No	Possible
Well-demarcated border	Yes	No	Yes	No	Yes
Markedly itchy	No	Yes	Possible	Possible	No
Symmetrical	Yes	Yes	No	Possible	No
Severe dandruff	Possible	Possible	Possible	Yes	No

Possible investigations

LIKELY: none.

POSSIBLE: Wood's light, skin scrapings/hair samples, patch testing.

SMALL PRINT: skin biopsy, syphilis serology, FBC, ESR/CRP, fasting glucose or HbA1c.

- Green fluorescence under UV (Wood's) light is diagnostic of microsporum fungal infection.
- Skin scrapings and hair samples for mycology: will help differentiate fungal infections from similar rashes.
- Skin biopsy: may be the only way to achieve a firm diagnosis in obscure rashes, and is essential if malignancy suspected.
- Patch testing: to establish the likely allergen in allergic contact eczema.
- Syphilis serology: if justified by clinical features or obscure pattern.
- FBC and ESR/CRP: may suggest significant underlying disease (e.g. T-cell lymphoma); ESR/CRP also elevated in Reiter's disease.
- Fasting glucose or HbA1c: check for diabetes in recurrent fungal infections.

TOP TIPS

- To help distinguish between fungal and eczematous rashes, look at the symmetry and edges of the lesions. Fungal rashes are usually asymmetrical with a scaly, raised edge.
- In the presence of a fungal rash, look for infection elsewhere (e.g. groins and feet) and treat both areas, otherwise the problem is likely to recur.
- In uncertain cases, explain to the patient that the real diagnosis may only become apparent as the rash develops (the typical example being the herald patch of pityriasis rosea looking like initially tinea corporis) – invite the patient to return for reassessment if your initial treatment proves unsuccessful.
- A symmetrical, glazed, scaly and fissured rash on the soles of a trainer-loving child or adolescent is juvenile plantar dermatosis.
- Eight per cent of people with psoriasis will have arthropathy, which is usually also associated with nail changes. Check the nails and ask about joint symptoms in patients with psoriasis.

☑ Erythroderma – universal redness and scaling caused, rarely, by psoriasis, eczema, mycosis fungoides and drug eruptions – renders the patient systemically unwell. Urgent inpatient treatment is required.

☑ A solitary, well-defined, slowly growing scaly plaque on the face, hands or legs of the middle-aged or elderly patient is probably Bowen's disease – but it can easily be mistaken for an isolated patch of eczema or psoriasis.

☑ If a pityriasis rosea-like rash extends to the palms and soles, with fever, malaise, sore throat and lymphadenopathy, consider secondary syphilis.

NOTES:

URINARY

Blood in urine

Excessive urination

Frequency

Incontinence

Nocturia

Retention

BLOOD IN URINE

The GP overview

Bright red blood in the urine causes instant alarm in a patient, and usually generates an emergency appointment or an out-of-hours call. Blood may also be picked up by dipstick testing or MSU during the assessment of some other problem or in a routine medical. This is often less frightening even when disclosed to the patient, but should prompt full investigation.

Differential diagnosis

COMMON
- UTI
- bladder tumour
- renal/ureteric stones
- urethritis
- prostatic hypertrophy/carcinoma of prostate

OCCASIONAL
- jogging and hard exercise
- renal carcinoma
- chronic interstitial cystitis
- anticoagulant therapy
- nephritis/glomerulonephritis

RARE
- renal tuberculosis
- polycystic kidney disease
- blood dyscrasias: thrombocytopenia, haemophilia, sickle-cell disease
- infective endocarditis
- schistosomiasis (common abroad)
- trauma

Ready reckoner

	UTI	Bladder tumour	Stones	Urethritis	Prostate
Frank blood	Possible	Possible	Possible	No	Possible
Dysuria	Yes	No	Yes	Yes	No
Urethral discharge	No	No	No	Yes	No
Poor urinary stream	No	Possible	Possible	No	Yes
Loin pain	Possible	No	Possible	No	No

Possible investigations

LIKELY: urinalysis, MSU, FBC, U&E, ACR/PCR.

POSSIBLE: PSA, ultrasound, plain abdominal X-ray, IVU, cystoscopy.

SMALL PRINT: urethral swab, CT scan, urine cytology, renal biopsy, angiography.

- Urinalysis: pus cells and nitrite in UTI. Pus cells alone in urethritis, TB and bladder tumour. Presence of protein suggests renal disease.
- Urine microscopy and culture to establish pathogen in infection. May show casts in renal disease.
- FBC and U&E help establish basic renal function and any associated anaemia or leucocytosis; consider PSA – usually elevated in prostatic carcinoma.
- ACR/PCR: to quantify any proteinuria.
- Urethral swabs if urethritis (best done at GUM clinic).
- If painless haematuria, ultrasound may show renal tumour or polycystic kidneys; CT may be more useful.
- IVU is investigation of choice if renal/ureteric stones are suspected (when pain is present); plain abdominal X-ray useful when attack has settled (reveals 90% of stones). IVU also required if ultrasound, abdominal X-ray and cystoscopy are all negative.
- Specialist investigations include cystoscopy, urinary cytology, renal biopsy and angiography.

TOP TIPS

- Microscopic haematuria in an asymptomatic menstruating woman can be ignored temporarily; repeat the urinalysis at mid-cycle.
- Remember that there are other less common causes of spurious haematuria – sometimes the blood may be coming from the rectum or vagina. Assess each case carefully and be prepared to rethink if symptoms persist but urological investigations prove negative.
- Some food pigments, beetroot and certain drugs (e.g. nitrofurantoin) can colour the urine red – confirm haematuria with urinalysis to save the patient unnecessary tests.

- Painless frank haematuria is an ominous sign indicating possible malignancy.
- Beware of recent onset of recurrent cystitis with haematuria in the elderly. The underlying cause may be a bladder tumour, especially if the haematuria (micro- or macroscopic) does not settle with treatment of the infection.
- Renal tumours can sometimes present with renal colic, as blood clots in the ureters mimic the effects of stones. A useful clue is that the bleeding may precede the pain.
- Haematuria requires emergency admission if there is significant blood loss or clot retention.

NOTES:

EXCESSIVE URINATION

The GP overview

Polyuria is a highly subjective symptom and one which presents rather less often than urinary frequency (which is dealt with separately, see p. 416). Most of the causes of polyuria listed here are also, by implication, causes of polydipsia – the only causes of true polydipsia not included are those due to dehydration.

Differential diagnosis

COMMON
- diabetes mellitus (DM)
- diuretic therapy
- chronic renal failure (CRF)
- hypercalcaemia (e.g. osteoporosis treatment, multiple bony metastases, hyperparathyroidism)
- alcohol

OCCASIONAL
- potassium depletion: chronic diarrhoea, diuretics, primary hyperaldosteronism
- relief of chronic urinary obstruction
- drugs: lithium carbonate, demeclocycline, amphotericin B, glibenclamide, gentamicin
- cranial diabetes insipidus (hypothalamo-pituitary tumour, skull trauma, sarcoidosis or histiocytosis X)
- Cushing's disease from excessive corticosteroid doses and ACTH-secreting bronchial carcinoma
- sickle-cell anaemia
- early chronic pyelonephritis

RARE
- psychogenic polydipsia (compulsive water drinking)
- supraventricular tachycardia
- DIDMOAD syndrome (diabetes insipidus, diabetes mellitus, optic atrophy, deafness: autosomal recessive)
- familial cranial diabetes insipidus (autosomal dominant inheritance)
- familial nephrogenic diabetes insipidus (males only: X-linked recessive)
- Fanconi syndrome

Ready reckoner

	DM	Diuretic therapy	CRF	Alcohol	High Ca^{2+}
Marked thirst	Yes	No	No	No	Yes
Other abnormalities on urinalysis	Possible	No	Possible	No	No
Abdominal pain and vomiting	Possible	No	No	No	Yes
Episodic	No	Possible	No	Yes	No
Anorexia/weight loss	Yes	No	Possible	No	Possible

Possible investigations

LIKELY: urinalysis, fasting glucose or HbA1c.

POSSIBLE: FBC, U&E, serum calcium.

SMALL PRINT: blood film, further specialist investigations (see below).

- Urinalysis: glucose and possible ketones in diabetes; possible haematuria and proteinuria with renal problems; specific gravity very low in diabetes insipidus and psychogenic polydipsia.
- Fasting glucose or HbA1c: to confirm diabetes mellitus.
- FBC: normochromic anaemia in CRF; film for sickle-cell anaemia.
- U&E: to detect potassium deficiency and abnormalities suggesting CRF.
- Serum calcium: elevated in hypercalcaemia.
- Further specialist investigations: many of the aforementioned 'causes' will need further investigation in secondary care to establish underlying aetiology (e.g. ultrasound and renal biopsy in CRF, water deprivation test for diabetes insipidus, CT scan if possible pituitary lesion, and so on).

TOP TIPS

- Take time to clarify the symptoms. It is essential to differentiate polyuria from frequency, as the causes are very different.
- Remember alcohol as a possible cause, especially in young males. Patients can be surprisingly slow to make quite obvious connections.
- Refer for more detailed investigation if the symptoms are clear-cut and baseline tests draw a blank.

☑ Diabetes mellitus is not the only cause of polyuria with thirst. If urinalysis is negative for sugar, consider diabetes insipidus or hypercalcaemia.

☑ Weight loss and cough in a smoker with polyuria suggests a possible ACTH-secreting tumour. Arrange an urgent CXR.

☑ If urinalysis reveals glucose and ketones in a known or new diabetic, arrange for urgent assessment with a view to admission for stabilisation.

☑ Renal disease is likely in patients with polydipsia who have blood and protein on urinalysis.

NOTES:

FREQUENCY

The GP overview

This means an increased frequency of micturition, and is usually associated with the passage of small amounts of urine. It is not the same as increased production of urine (see Excessive urination, p. 413). It is a commonly presented problem, affecting women far more often than men: the average GP will deal with around 60 cases of cystitis (the main cause) each year. Terminology can be confusing – we now use 'LUTS' for what we used to describe as 'prostatism'.

Differential diagnosis

COMMON

- infective cystitis
- anxiety
- overactive bladder syndrome
- bladder calculus
- lower urinary tract symptoms (LUTS) in men

OCCASIONAL

- interstitial cystitis (non-infective)
- prostatitis
- pregnancy
- ureteric calculus (in lower third of ureter precipitates reflex frequency)
- urethritis, pyelonephritis
- iatrogenic (e.g. diuretics)
- bladder neck hypertrophy
- 'habit frequency'

RARE

- pelvic space-occupying lesion, e.g. fibroid, ovarian cyst, carcinoma
- secondary to pelvic inflammation: PID, appendicitis, diverticulitis, adjacent tumour
- bladder tumour (benign or malignant)
- post-radiotherapy fibrosis (testicular, ovarian and prostatic cancer)
- tuberculous cystitis/renal TB
- fibrosis secondary to chronic sepsis from long-term catheter drainage

Ready reckoner

	Anxiety	Infective cystitis	Overactive bladder syndrome	LUTS	Bladder calculus
Dysuria	No	Yes	No	No	Possible
Eased when prone	No	No	No	No	Yes
Hesitancy, slow flow	No	No	No	Yes	Possible
Nocturnal frequency	No	Yes	Yes	Possible	No
Abnormal urinalysis	No	Yes	No	Possible	Yes

Possible investigations

LIKELY: urinalysis, MSU, urinary frequency volume chart.

POSSIBLE: urethral swab, PSA, uroflowmetry, urodynamic studies, plain abdominal X-ray, IVU, cystoscopy, CA-125.

SMALL PRINT: pelvic ultrasound, U&E, pregnancy test and three EMUs for TB.

- ⬛ Urinalysis: protein, nitrites, leucocytes and possible haematuria in infection; possible stone or tumour if blood alone.
- ⬛ MSU: microscopy may show abnormal epithelial cells, blood, pus and help identify pathogen in infection.
- ⬛ Urinary frequency volume chart – may be useful in men with LUTS.
- ⬛ Swab any urethral discharge present for *Chlamydia* and gonorrhoea.
- ⬛ CA-125 – may be useful if ovarian cancer suspected.
- ⬛ EMU: for pregnancy test; also three EMUs to check for TB if suspected (e.g. sterile pyuria).
- ⬛ U&E: check if assessment suggests chronic sepsis or outflow obstruction.
- ⬛ PSA: consider this if LUTS in male.
- ⬛ Specialist tests include: uroflowmetry (for LUTS, urodynamic studies (for unstable bladder), IVU and cystoscopy (for stones and tumours) and ultrasound (for pelvic masses or if CA-125 elevated).

TOP TIPS

- ⬛ Frequency due to anxiety is typically long term, worse with stress and cold weather, and is associated with a normal urinalysis.
- ⬛ It is reasonable to make an empirical diagnosis of overactive bladder syndrome in a non-pregnant female with frequency in whom CA-125, pelvic examination and urinalysis are entirely normal.
- ⬛ An unrecognised pregnancy may present with frequency: ask about periods, and do a pregnancy test if a period has been missed.

☑ In the elderly, a bladder tumour may present as cystitis. If a new, recurring problem, or haematuria attributed to the cystitis does not settle with antibiotics, consider referral.

☑ Do not ignore sterile pyuria on the MSU: possible causes include urethritis and TB.

☑ The adult patient with frequency who has persistent microscopic haematuria but no other abnormalities on urinalysis may have a stone or tumour. Refer.

☑ Appendicitis can cause mild frequency and pyuria. Do not be misled by the urinalysis into an inappropriate diagnosis of UTI: act according to the clinical findings.

☑ UTI in infancy is a major cause of renal failure. Manage according to NICE guidance.

NOTES:

INCONTINENCE

The GP overview

Incontinence is involuntary micturition. It is not a common presenting symptom, embarrassment tending to inhibit patients, but it is often mentioned as a 'while I'm here' or noted by the doctor, typically because of the characteristic odour when visiting an elderly patient. It may present more frequently in the future as the problem receives more publicity and patients realise that help is available. The population prevalence in women is around 10%, but is probably much higher in older age groups.

Differential diagnosis

COMMON
- stress incontinence (with or without prolapse)
- infective cystitis
- overactive bladder syndrome: idiopathic or secondary to other problems, e.g. CVA, dementia, Parkinson's disease
- chronic outflow obstruction, e.g. prostatic enlargement, bladder neck stenosis, urethral stenosis
- after prostatectomy (usually temporary)

OCCASIONAL
- chronic UTI
- interstitial cystitis
- bladder stone or tumour
- after abdomino-pelvic surgery and radiotherapy
- fistula: vesicovaginal/uterine, ureterovaginal (surgery and malignancy)
- polyuria (any cause, e.g. diabetes, diuretics – particularly if compounded by immobility in the elderly)

RARE
- after pelvic fracture (direct sphincter damage with or without neurological damage)
- congenital abnormalities: short urethra, wide urethra, epispadias, ectopic ureter
- sensory neuropathy, e.g. diabetes and syphilis
- multiple sclerosis, syringomyelia
- paraplegia, cauda equina lesion
- psychogenic

Ready reckoner

	Stress incontinence	Infective cystitis	Overactive bladder syndrome	Outflow obstruction	Prostatectomy
Stress pattern	Yes	No	No	Possible	Possible
Urge pattern	No	Yes	Yes	No	Yes
Overflow pattern	No	No	No	Yes	No
Dysuria	No	Yes	No	No	Possible
Palpable bladder	No	No	No	Yes	No

Possible investigations

LIKELY: urinalysis, MSU.

POSSIBLE: PSA, U&E, ultrasound, IVU, urodynamic studies, uroflowmetry.

SMALL PRINT: fasting sugar or HbA1c blood sugar, syphilis serology, cystoscopy, neurological investigations.

- Urinalysis: to test for infection and diabetes.
- MSU: to confirm infection and guide antibiotic treatment.
- Fasting sugar or HbA1c and syphilis serology: if diabetes or syphilis a possible cause of neuropathy.
- PSA: consider this if LUTS or prostatic enlargement on examination.
- U&E: to assess renal function in chronic outflow obstruction.
- Ultrasound good for assessing renal size non-invasively: may suggest outflow obstruction or chronic infection.
- IVU best for looking for renal scarring of chronic UTI, structural anomalies and demonstrating residual urine; may also reveal site of outflow obstruction and fistulae.
- Specialist investigations may include: urodynamic studies (helpful to distinguish between urge and stress incontinence), uroflowmetry (prostatism), cystoscopy (may reveal cause of outflow obstruction, stone or tumour) and neurological investigations (e.g. imaging of spinal cord).

TOP TIPS

- Incontinence has many causes, but can often be broadly categorised into one of three groups: stress incontinence (e.g. with coughing), urge incontinence ('when I've got to go, I've got to go') and continuous, like water over the edge of a dam (e.g. through a vesicovaginal fistula, or in overflow from a chronically distended bladder).
- The aetiology may be multifactorial, particularly in the elderly. Mobility, vision, distance to the toilet and ongoing medication may all be relevant.
- Overactive bladder syndrome and stress incontinence can be difficult to distinguish. The

latter rarely causes nocturnal incontinence, while it may be a feature of overactive bladder syndrome. If in doubt, refer for urodynamic studies.

- Adopt a sympathetic approach. Incontinence can have a devastating impact on self-esteem and seriously affect a patient's social and sexual functioning.

- Incontinence with saddle anaesthesia and leg weakness suggests a cauda equina lesion. This is a neurological emergency: refer urgently.
- Continuous incontinence suggests significant pathology, such as a fistula, chronic outflow obstruction or a neurological problem.
- Never empty the huge bladder of chronic retention in one go. This can cause bleeding and renal complications. Admit for catheterisation and controlled release.
- Adult-onset nocturnal enuresis suggests chronic retention.

NOTES:

NOCTURIA

The GP overview

Nocturia may present in isolation or it may be a manifestation of other urinary disturbances such as polyuria or frequency. Surprisingly, in older age groups, it is as common in women as men. Occasional nocturia is, of course, quite normal – the symptom should only be viewed as pathological when it causes disruption or distress.

Differential diagnosis

COMMON
- age related (in part caused by a reduction in bladder capacity)
- excess fluid at bed time (especially alcohol)
- any cause of swollen ankles (the recumbent posture redistributes the fluid load at night) – see Swollen ankles, p. 312
- cystitis
- LUTS

OCCASIONAL
- overactive bladder syndrome
- lower urinary tract obstruction (other than prostate problems)
- any other cause of urinary frequency (see Frequency, p. 416)
- diabetes mellitus
- any other cause of polyuria (see Excessive urination, p. 413)
- sleep apnoea (causes overproduction of urine)

RARE
- anxiety
- drug side effect (rare because drugs likely to cause a diuresis are usually taken in the morning)
- diabetes insipidus

Ready reckoner

	Age related	Excess fluid	Swollen ankles	Cystitis	LUTS
Daytime ankle oedema	Possible	No	Yes	No	No
Daytime frequency	Possible	No	No	Yes	Possible
Poor urinary flow	No	No	No	No	Yes
Long-term problem	Yes	Possible	Yes	No	Yes
Polyuria	No	Yes	Yes	No	No

Possible investigations

NOTE: urinary frequency, polyuria, or swollen ankles as 'causes' of nocturia will need investigating in their own right – see the relevant sections for more details on each of these topics.

LIKELY: urinalysis, MSU, urinary frequency volume chart.

POSSIBLE: blood sugar, PSA.

SMALL PRINT: cystoscopy, urodynamic studies, IVP/ultrasound, water deprivation test.

- Urinalysis: protein, nitrites, leucocytes and possible haematuria in infection; glucose in diabetes; specific gravity very low in diabetes insipidus.
- MSU: to confirm infection and identify pathogen.
- Urinary frequency volume chart – to help distinguish nocturnal polyuria (increased urine production at night) from reduced bladder storage capacity.
- Blood sugar: to confirm diabetes mellitus.
- PSA: pros and cons of this test may be discussed if assessment raises the possibility of prostate cancer.
- Specialist tests include: cystoscopy and IVU/ultrasound (for lower urinary tract obstruction), urodynamic studies (for unstable bladder) and water deprivation test (for diabetes insipidus).

TOP TIPS

- In the elderly, the cause is often multifactorial.
- The effects – such as disturbed sleep, a disrupted household, exhaustion and occasional incontinence – may be more important to the patient than the specific diagnosis.
- Swollen ankles – of any aetiology – are frequently overlooked as an underlying cause.
- Nocturia may just be a manifestation (albeit the most distressing) of polyuria or urinary frequency. Focus your approach on the underlying problem.

- Exclude diabetes – but remember that it is not the only cause of polyuria, nocturia and thirst.
- A habitual 'nightcap' may be the cause of nocturia – and may be a pointer to an underlying alcohol problem, especially in solitary elderly males.

NOTES:

RETENTION

The GP overview

Retention is failure to empty the bladder completely. The acute form characteristically affects men, presents urgently and requires immediate catheterisation or hospitalisation. Chronic retention may produce few symptoms and may only be discovered during palpation of the abdomen.

Differential diagnosis

COMMON

- prostatic hypertrophy: benign, rarely carcinoma
- anticholinergic drugs: bladder stabilisers and tricyclic antidepressants
- constipation
- bladder neck obstruction/urethral stricture
- UTI (including prostatitis and prostatic abscess)

OCCASIONAL

- urethral calculus
- 'holding on' (leads to prostatic congestion)
- pelvic mass: retroverted, gravid uterus or fibroid uterus
- acute genital herpes (via local inflammation and interference with neurological control of detrusor reflex arc)
- clot retention (e.g. after bleed from tumour or post-TURP bleed)
- balanoposthitis in children (if very painful)

RARE

- neurological: MS, syphilis, spinal cord compression
- pedunculated bladder tumour
- traumatic rupture of urethra
- foreign body inserted into anterior urethra
- phimosis
- psychological

Ready reckoner

	Prostatic hypertrophy	Drugs	Constipation	Bladder neck	UTI
Enlarged prostate PR	Yes	No	No	No	Possible
Acute	Possible	Yes	Possible	No	Yes
Young patient	No	Possible	No	Possible	Possible
Abnormal urinalysis	Possible	No	No	No	Yes
Palpable colon	No	No	Yes	No	No

Possible investigations

LIKELY: urinalysis, MSU.

POSSIBLE: U&E, PSA, ultrasound, IVU, cystoscopy.

SMALL PRINT: neurological investigations, prostatic biopsy, urethrography (all hospital-based investigations).

- Urinalysis of any urine available may confirm a UTI as the cause; may also reveal microscopic haematuria if a stone or bladder tumour.
- MSU: will confirm infective agent in UTI.
- U&E: renal failure may follow chronic retention.
- PSA may be worth considering if preceding symptoms of prostatism or abnormal prostate on examination.
- Specialist tests may include: renal ultrasound (reveals obstruction and pelvic masses), IVU (may reveal site of obstruction and will provide information about renal function), cystoscopy (may be diagnostic and therapeutic for stones, stricture, bladder outflow obstruction and bladder tumour), neurological investigations (e.g. spinal cord imaging if cord lesion suspected), prostatic biopsy (if suspicious area of prostate palpable) and urethrography (for stricture).

TOP TIPS

- Do not overlook faecal impaction in the elderly patient as a cause of urinary retention.
- 'First-aid' relief of retention when the cause is a painful perineal condition (e.g. balanoposthitis, herpes simplex or UTI) may be achieved by encouraging the patient to urinate while immersed in a warm bath.
- Anuria can be mistaken for retention. A straightforward clinical assessment should differentiate the two conditions.

☑ A history suggesting a disc prolapse with urinary retention indicates possible cord compression – admit immediately.

☑ Sudden stoppage of urine with a pain like a blow to the bladder and passage of a few drops of blood is pathognomic of urethral calculus.

☑ Beware of any drugs with anticholinergic side effects in patients with a history of outflow obstruction – they may precipitate acute retention.

☑ Avoid catheterisation when sepsis is likely (e.g. possible UTI) – instrumentation may result in septicaemia. Instead, admit to hospital for catheterisation under appropriate antibiotic cover.

☑ Do not catheterise the patient with chronic retention; admit for controlled drainage. Sudden decompression can result in haematuria and renal complications.

NOTES:

INDEX

CPD with Radcliffe

You can now use a selection of our books to achieve CPD (Continuing Professional Development) points through directed reading.

We provide a free online form and downloadable certificate for your appraisal portfolio. Look for the CPD logo and register with us at: www.radcliffehealth.com/cpd